THE PHYSICIAN WITHIN YOU

THE PHYSICIAN WITHIN YOU

Medicine for the Millennium

Gladys Taylor McGarey, M.D., M.D. (H)
with Jess Stearn

Inkwell Productions
Scottsdale, Arizona
www.selfpublishing.com

ISBN 0-9658158-5-4

Published By:
INKWELL PRODUCTIONS
3370 N. Hayden Road #123-276
Scottsdale, Arizona 85251
Telephone: (480) 315-9636
Fax: (480) 315-9641
www.selfpublishing.com

Cover Design by:
COMPOSING ARTS
Scottsdale, Arizona
(480) 423-8858

Printed by:
BILTMORE PRO PRINT
Phoenix, Arizona

Developed by:
SELFPUBLISHING.COM
www.selfpublishing.com

A portion of the proceeds of this book will benefit the Gladys Taylor
McGarey Medical Foundation. This is a non-profit organization which
furthers the cause of integrative medicine through education and
research about the mind-body-spirit connection in healing.

CONTENTS

PREFACE

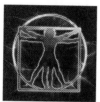 This book tells the real stories of real people, their living experiences as they have enriched my life and as I have influenced theirs.

This book is for all people, physicians and patients alike. There is no physician who, at one time or another, will not be a patient and each of us has within us that divine spark which we have chosen to call "the physician within."

There have been times when I have worked with a patient who had a bleeding peptic ulcer. The surgeon and I would remove the offending part of the stomach and bring about a cure but if that is all that we did, there would not be a true healing. We needed to get to the basis of why they got sick in the first place and if we did not, the problem would be back perhaps at an even deeper and more severe level. We could have cured the disease but not had a healing of the patient—not without bringing forth the physician within.

Our purpose in writing this book is to help physicians and patients alike to work together in awakening the physician within, empowering our divine selves to not only bring healing to ourselves but to our beautiful planet. We are all a part of the whole and as each of us takes responsibility for our own healing, we are all made a little better.

So join me and we will travel together on an adventure in healing the whole person.

ACKNOWLEDGMENTS

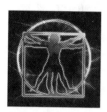 I gratefully acknowledge the patients who shared their stories in this book, and the many others who helped me learn about the amazing dynamics of body/mind/spirit connections in healing. I also want to honor my colleagues, the physicians who work as partners with patients and help them take responsibility for wielding the keys to the remarkable healing power inherent in each human being.

I am thankful for the wisdom shared by many indigenous people and the teachers and angels who guided me along the path of learning. My thanks to those early pioneers who helped open the doors of knowledge in holistic medicine. They include: Edgar Cayce, Hugh Lynn Cayce, Charles Thomas Cayce, Elisabeth Kubler-Ross, M.D., Rachel Naomi Remen, M.D., Larry Dossey, M.D., Carl Taylor, M.D., and many others who contributed to the field of mind/body medicine. Due to space limitations, I can't include the names of many important individuals who have shared their insight and knowledge. I'm sure you know who you are. Please accept my thanks.

This work evolved largely due to the expert journalistic skills and hard work of Jess Stearn.

I also wish to thank Nick Ligidakis, who made the publishing of this book possible.

Heartfelt appreciation goes to the foundation's executive director, Fern Stewart Welch, C.M.A., and the staff. Thanks also to other foundation members, such as Jerome A. Landau and Carol Osman Brown. These marvelous individuals helped carry the vision of this book and gave greatly of their time and efforts in facilitating the writing, editing and proofing of the manuscript.

I also wish to thank my six children for their continuing support of my work, and especially my daughter, Helene Wechsler, M.D., M.D.(H), who adds great joy to my continuing work as a family physician.

INTRODUCTION

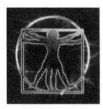 Some 20 years ago, a hardy band of physicians met at a desert retreat in California to discuss what was wrong with the practice of medicine in this country—and what could be done about it. I was one of that tiny band of five.

We were all painfully aware that medicine wasn't doing its best for the patient. Yet that was what medicine was all about: the patient. We also knew that there were physicians across the country, like ourselves, who were involved in various alternative aspects of medicine that were conventionally frowned upon, but which we believed were important and necessary. As practicing physicians, we not only felt restricted in our patient care. We were also concerned that a narrowing focus on the patient was just the beginning of what was wrong in conventional medicine. Humankind was much more than body/mind. The spirit and the aspirations, the fears and the deep longings of the patient needed to be addressed before any true healing could be accomplished.

Our beliefs had no place in the teachings of the medical schools and the hospitals, or in the way conventional medicine was being practiced in its unimaginative and dogmatic manner. Nowhere did we see any emphasis on what the patient cared about.

Insurance companies and Medicare were having an increasing and detrimental influence on the way medicine was being practiced, and the patient-physician relationship was no longer the primary focus. In the past, the first words a new patient heard were usually, "How can I help you?" or "What is troubling you?" Then the prevailing question became, "What insurance do you have?" If the patient was elderly, the question often was, "What insurance do you have besides Medicare?" As for Medicare, it was telling doctors how many times a week we could see patients, no matter how ill they were, without putting them into the hospital, when that was the last place they should be.

Physicians, like other people, have families to support and children to educate. But our band of five, sharing this problem, saw that money all too often influenced the relationships between patient and doctor. The emphasis was all wrong. Our primary job as doctors was to help the patients help themselves by getting them involved in their own healing, and by working on the person more than the disease. We thought of this as (w)holistic medicine. It encompassed all safe modalities, diagnoses and treatments, including drugs and surgery, and it looked closely at the whole person and their lifestyle: physical, nutritional, environmental, emotional and spiritual.

When we let other doctors around the country know what we were up to, they rallied around the cause of a patient-first organization such as we envisioned. In 1978, at a meeting of 300 physicians in Denver, we formed the American Holistic Medical Association. Dr. Norman Shealy, a prominent neurosurgeon, was our first president. I was vice president, and subsequently succeeded him.

As a burgeoning group we soon discovered that we were not alone. While the usual "good old boys" continued to look down their noses at a less conventional medicine, the idea took hold among many other open-minded physicians, swelling interest in holistic and alternative medicine, and even leading to the establishment of a Department of Alternative Medicine at the National Institutes of Health in Washington, D.C.

Early on we decided that even though we were dealing with the whole person, we should spell "holistic" with an "h" because we were essentially working with the spirit of people, and *holistic* was derived from the word *holy* or spiritual.

Many of us are confused about what medicine is. In medical school we're taught that it is a science. Yet I truly believe that medicine is an art, and science is a magnificent tool used in that art. An art is hard to teach and hard to control because each artist brings his or her own creative spirit and personality to it.

Science needs to be controlled and needs to have parameters. And because we think medicine is a science, we are constantly trying to control it, to make physicians and patients fit into a particular category or a particular model. We've made a god out of science, and its temples are hospitals, medical schools, scientific laboratories and even the government. There is nothing wrong with any of these except that our perception of them is all out of proportion. We think that unless a therapeutic modality comes down from one of these institutions to the physician or to the public, it is not "scientific."

The science of medicine deals with the study of disease, which is a deadly process. The art of medicine deals with the study of life, which is a healthy process, filled with joy. Physicians need to look at the patient as a partner. Patients need to have something to say about their own healing. In the art of medicine, the human body is the temple.

We need to create a whole new model of health care where holistic and conventional practices are brought together for the good of both the patient and the physician. The medicine of the future, as I envision it, will integrate the spiritual dimension of healing and acknowledge the spiritual nature of humankind. Then true inner healing can happen. Without this, it is possible for the physical body to be cured, but a true, lasting healing cannot be fully realized.

I see patient care of the future revolving around a center where people of all races and conditions come for healing in a setting where like-minded practitioners (allopaths, homeopathics, chiropractors, psychologists, and physical and biofeedback therapists), together with shamans and healers of all cultures, respect one another's abilities and work individually or together to help the most important people of all—patients—to heal themselves.

To Be a Doctor

Give us enough work to do,
And strength enough to
do the work.

—RUDYARD KIPLING
A Doctor's Work

I was two years old, barely able to speak, and yet I knew I had come into this life to be a physician, just as my daughter, Helene, would later know. (Perhaps this is why today we are partners in our own practice.) Both my parents were physicians, and this likely had something to do with my decision, but not totally, since only one of my four siblings became a doctor. It had to be an inner knowing, an awareness that I was born with. What the Hindus, with whom I was raised, call

1

dharma, a cosmic principle defining the different nature of all God's creatures.

My parents were medical missionaries in the Presbyterian church. They worked together on the bleak southern slopes of the Himalayan mountains and in the dark steamy jungles rife with malaria and ferocious animals, mending the bodies and spirits of impoverished natives who looked on them as ministering angels. I spoke Hindustani, the language of my ayah, my nursemaid, before I spoke English. When my parents were in the villages, working in tents or out in the open with patients who flocked to see them, we children, my three brothers, my sister and I, were in and out and all around. Being with the sick and getting them to relax and feel comfortable was as natural to me as breathing.

I never doubted why my down-to-earth Midwestern parents gave their lives to these simple people in this remote and often dangerous land. When I saw the glow of gratitude and love in the misty eyes of children and grown-ups who were clad in tattered and makeshift clothes, I understood why my parents did this work. Since my parents made no secret of the fact that they were also Christian ministers, the people they helped were often interested in the God they served and in this Jesus who had some vague connection in their minds to a universal God so like their own.

I mingled with the Hindu and Moslem children as if they were my own family. Some of these relationships have continued to this day. I was an active, involved child, an adventurous Sagittarius always nosing around to see what was going on. I would sometimes sing hymns at our services in the shadows of the towering mountains, or in the jungle villages, where a tiger or a leopard might poke his head in a tent, and then, luckily, drift off. As a child one of my favorite hymns was the candle song.

Jesus bids us shine with a clear, pure light,
Like a little candle burning in the night.
In this world of darkness we must shine,
You in your corner and I in mine.

I also tried it in Hindustani, but of course it didn't rhyme as well.

I was practicing medicine even then, conventional jungle and mountain medicine, helping my mom and dad to bind up splintered arms and legs, and doling out the quinine for the malaria which almost everybody, including us, came down with. At this time, already envisioning myself a doctor, I noted the one unvarying constant in all healings, whether it was a broken leg or a case of leprosy: the tender, loving care my parents gave each patient, the kind word, the touch of a hand, the reassuring embrace.

My concept of healing and of the physician within started back in this strange and compelling land. I knew then that we who aspired to be doctors had special work to do and special tools with which to do that work. It was a matter of searching within ourselves to find and to work with those tools. As I look back, the concept of the physician within reminds me of the candle I loved to sing about. Every one of us has this candle which shines with a clear, pure light, but sometimes the light gets cloudy, or almost blows out, or the candle runs out of wax. So many different things can happen to the light, like they do in our own lives, when the wind blows too hard, or we get too close to the flame.

The patient is also like the candle. We, the physicians, I see now, are there to keep the light shining bright. When it flickers or dims we help trim the wick, curb the draft, renew the wax. We must keep our own light clear and pure to be the keepers of that flame. Ours is a noble profession. How well I realized this as I saw my parents work from the break of dawn to dusk treating the patients who streamed into our camp. Some were so sick they had to be carried. Others, faltering and barely able to see, sat patiently as my father performed the surgery they needed and sent them happily on their way. And my mother worked valiantly at his side, applying dressings to running sores and gaping wounds. Each of them chattered pleasantly with the patients in their native tongue as they made them comfortable and relieved their fears.

My young eyes noted the changes in the people, the hope and the relief coming into their faces. And I knew more than ever that this was what I had come to do and needed to do. I was never happier than when I was helping apply a dressing or making the infirm and elderly comfortable. As a child of six, I became furious with an English classmate who asked what I was going to be when I grew up. It was not an unusual question for a first-grader, but my reply was unusual.

"I'm going to be a doctor," I said.

The girl laughed and said with a smirk, "You can't be a doctor. Men are doctors. Women are nurses."

I guess she didn't know about my mother, or my Aunt Belle, who was taking care of lepers in a nearby colony. I was so mad I didn't speak to my classmate for weeks. Finally, when she opened a conversation with me, the first thing I said was, "You know, I'm still going to be a doctor. And you can be a nurse, if you like."

Our parents made sure that we went to the best school available in the area, a nondenominational school established for the children of missionaries. It was taken for granted that we would finish our higher education in the homeland and then have the option to stay in the States or return to India.

We went to the Woodstock School on the southern slopes of the Himalayas in the town of Landour, Mussoorie. My father,

John Taylor, got a kick out of this since he grew up on a Kansas farm and had gone to medical school in Missouri. There he met and married another student, Elizabeth Siehl, my mother. Now he joked about the name Mussoorie, saying it almost made him feel at home.

Classes at the Woodstock School ran from mid-March through November. Every morning we had to walk a mile from our home in the Himalayas to the school, and then walk the mile back in the afternoon. Our home was 8,000 feet above sea level and the school stood at 7,000 feet. It was easy going downhill, somewhat more difficult going uphill. We never minded climbing the hill when we were going home, and this was my first insight into the power of a strong incentive—in this case, going home. During the monsoon season the rains would wash away what passed for roads. We'd be drenched going to school and have to hang up our outer clothes to dry in the classroom.

In November, when school recessed, we'd move from the Himalayas to the plains where Mother and Dad had their winter work laid out for them. These were the best times of our lives. We traveled as a family with our parents, whom we looked up to and believed could do almost anything. We'd go from one village to the next in the dark jungles, staying a week or 10 days in each village before we packed our belongings and medical equipment in an ox cart and moved on. If nothing else, it taught us to be hardy and self-reliant, qualities continually stressed by my father.

There were times when we pitched camp beside the Ganges, India's sacred river, where it was great fun to swim if you stayed clear of the crocodiles and alligators who made it their home, and the snakes who came down to bathe on the river banks and quench their thirst. We were respectful of snakes, hoping they wouldn't bother us if we didn't bother them. Usually, they too had a healthy respect for the two-legged creature with the long stick—a high-powered rifle. From our camp we roamed through the villages at will, speaking the language like the natives, never feeling out of place. Quite often we would bring the smaller children home with us, back to our tent, if they looked particularly thin or hungry. This we did only with children of the poorest and lowest caste, the Untouchables. We whites were equally untouchable to the higher-caste Indians, who would not let their children eat any food contaminated by our touch. This experience stood me in good stead, for it was to make me bridle all my life at any racial or religious prejudice, seeing how self-limiting and unreasonable it was.

I came to love the Indian people, the common not-so-ordinary people, who never regarded us as outsiders. They saw how we took pains to know their language and live with them, and how my parents left their own land to help them. They could sense the interest and concern of these two unusual doctors who greeted them as equals and were so patient with each and every one regardless of caste.

I got to know the village people, the Indians, as well as I knew the whites. And there was much speculation in the villages about why and how we were white. Many had never seen a white person before, and one of the theories was that when we were born, our mothers wrapped us in white cotton which absorbed our natural color—a dusky brown, of course. I remember natives rubbing their hands over my face and bare arms and combing through my hair, marveling at how different they were from theirs.

We loved the winter months in the villages. I remember one particular campsite which was under a huge pepul tree, its trunk more than 40 feet around. We children built a tree house in its branches while our parents went about seeing patients.

My father and mother would see 200 patients a day, doing everything from pulling teeth and taking care of abscesses to dispensing medicine for malaria. There were no intensive care centers, no consultations, no referrals. Some natives even brought their sick and wounded animals. An elephant driver, a mahout, came in with a lame elephant. The poor animal was lumbering along in pain, groaning and moaning with each halting step. He had somehow gotten a bamboo spike through his leg and there was an open, draining sore. My father was off with my brothers hunting for game for the table. My mother had taken over the medical work while my older sister and I did what we could to help. The elephant reared up on his hind legs and trumpeted his protest as my mother probed the wound. Then she took a large syringe, filled it with a solution of potassium permanganate which I proudly handed to her, and speaking in a soothing voice, as though to an ordinary patient, she carefully syringed the ulcerated leg. The elephant thumped the ground, but my mother stood firm, talking to him all the while. As he quieted down she continued to inject the permanganate into one side of the leg, letting it drain out the other side. From time to time she looked up, catching her patient's eye and patting his leg gently. Somehow this seemed to calm him. She did this every day for a week, establishing a link between her patient—this wounded elephant—and herself, a caring physician. As his pain began to ease, the elephant became very devoted to her. He would follow my mother wherever she went. She would be doing something with a patient, then suddenly feel something circling her waist and look down to see the elephant's trunk—his idea of a fond embrace. Mother would smack his trunk and say, "Come now, be a nice boy," and he, being a gentleman, would desist. We children adopted the elephant and had wonderful rides on this grateful giant, who seemed to sense our connection with the woman who had healed him.

All this served as a lesson to me when years later, as a doctor, I recalled how this so-called lesser species had responded to the care and loving attention Mother had given him, and how she had instilled in him the trust that made the healing possible. Doctors don't have to love every patient, but they should love what they're doing with a patient. It helps. Take it from the elephant. The patient knows when a doctor cares, and it makes a difference.

There was another side to my parents' efforts. They had been sent out as missionaries not only to heal bodies and minds, but the human spirit. We would visit some homes with our Christian Bible, and share the stories of Jesus' miraculous healings. This was something the natives could relate to, particularly from people who were in the healing business.

There was never any pressure on my parents' part. My father thought it enough to expose the people to Jesus' message of love and salvation and let them take it from there. My parents believed in what they were doing and left what they couldn't do to the Lord. My father was not one to mince words. His message was clear to all of us: "Do what you can and take comfort that whatever the outcome, you gave it your best."

My father was equally clear about dealing with jungle life. We were brought up to be brave and hardy. "A faint heart," he would say, "never won anything."

Wild tigers, leopards, wolves and hyenas wandered into our camp, looking for a good meal. They weren't too fussy about who or what it was. They'd forage for cattle, peacocks and dogs, or pick off an occasional villager. Once a she-wolf approached the bed of one of the children, repeatedly coming back after being shooed away. She had lost one of her cubs and wanted to adopt one of ours. Life was often like that in India's jungles. My father hunted for game and to protect our settlement. As we grew into our teens, we also were expected to contribute to the safety of the community by hunting down the more dangerous animals. On a hunt one day, my father handed me a rifle and nodded into the thick of the jungle. I was 15 then, big and strong for my age. A spotted leopard came in view. My father nudged me, and raised his rifle, taking aim. I raised my rifle to my shoulder as I had seen my dad and brothers do. I took careful aim at this beautiful creature and fired at a spot about 10 feet over his head. My father's gun went off simultaneously. The leopard slumped to the ground. I drew in my breath. "You got him," my father said. He patted me on the shoulder. I knew my bullet hadn't killed the leopard. And so did my dad. He just wanted to let me know that it was all right. He understood.

In India, a doctor often had to improvise not only for his patients, but for his family, so they could stay alive and well. I learned early on about improvising by what was done to keep me alive and well.

The second-youngest of five children, I was the only one my mother didn't nurse because she had severe hemorrhaging at my birth. That presented the problem of feeding me. There were no baby bottles, nor for that matter any milk bottles, large or small, in that part of the country. My dad was not stumped for a moment. He went off to the village bazaar and came back with a toy tea kettle. He tied the end of a medicine dropper to the spout and poked a tiny hole in it. That was my milk bottle, from which I drank buffalo's milk.

During those days in India, in the late 1930s, virtually everybody had malaria. I was no exception. My malaria was complicated by a severe case of hepatitis and jaundice. I remember getting into my mother's diary one time and reading about the struggle they had had to keep me alive, and my own fight to survive, which would later make me acutely aware of what went through a patient's mind when death was close. I never realized how close I had come at the time, because my parents were calm and optimistic through it all. I still remember their prayers, positive and uplifting, and how they never visualized anything but my complete recovery. And there was always a hug and a smile. I have a feeling that their prayers, more than any rudimentary medicines, played a large part in my getting well. I believed that my parents, with their air of authority and command, could accomplish anything. And it was this kind of confidence that I later sought to inspire in my patients. My parents gave me the gift of thinking of myself as a well person having a transient bout with illness, and never as a sick person. I invariably use this experience of mine with patients who have seemed to let go of life. I let them know that the battle is not lost while there is something to live for.

From my first day in school, my heart was set on studying whatever I could to further my medical career. Yet it was hard parting from my parents when it was time to go off to America. "It will be a wonderful adventure," my mother assured me. I was only 16, and my parents, ever watchful for their young daughter, sent me off to a small college in New Concord, Ohio, near Cincinnati, where my mother's three sisters, retired teachers, lived. I didn't care much where I went as long as it prepared me for medical school, but I did realize for a quaking moment that it would be years before I saw my mother and dad again.

My two brothers and sister had preceded me to this college, a four-year undergraduate school with an interesting name— Muskingum College. It was a good school, as it turned out, and I had to work hard to catch up. I had no social life, I didn't feel like dating, and I had no clothing suitable for any social occasion, unless it was a super-dark movie house. I had worn my shoes down to where there were holes in the soles and I would put postcards in the bottom of them to keep my feet dry. I didn't consider any of this a hardship. My one single-minded goal was getting into medical school. Totally engrossed in my studies, I didn't have the time or inclination for anything else.

I was also struggling to get used to a formal white society, to the protocol, the customs, the prejudices, and to the drive of people to get ahead in a system that seemed painfully structured after my wide-ranging life in the Indian jungle. I was a curiosity on campus, a white girl from India. Students would brush by me or stare off when I caught their eye. I did make one or two friends, but they were a little offtrack like myself. It would have been nice, I remember thinking then, to fling away the shoes with the cardboard bottoms and stride off to class in my bare feet—not only for the comfort and freedom of it, but as a symbol of my free and independent spirit. As time passed I was no longer as much of an oddity, but it really made little difference to me anyway. I was so intent on being a doctor that anything removed from this goal was unimportant.

The years went by quickly and uneventfully. As I was finishing at Muskingum, I was still treading water, nervously awaiting acceptance into medical school. Finally, it came. A letter, which I read and reread a dozen times. I was accepted into Women's Medical School in Philadelphia.

I had no money for tuition, but I was able to get a scholarship from the Presbyterian Church with the understanding I would go back to India as a medical missionary, or pay the money back. To do this I had to join a presbytery, a division of the Presbyterian Church. My aunts were members of the Cincinnati Presbytery, so I arranged to join the presbytery there, little knowing at the time how this simple event would turn my life around.

While attending a church meeting, I sat down next to my aunts' minister, the only person I knew in the assemblage. Sitting in front of me, as it happened, was a good-looking young man who caught my eye. We exchanged glances. We were the only young people at the meeting. I had to stand up and tell why I was joining the presbytery. Then the young man stood up and told his story. It caught my interest. It turned out that he was the nephew of the pastor in whose church the meeting was being held. He said he was planning to be a minister. I, of course, had said I was planning to be a missionary. After the meeting he approached me and said he had a classmate at college from India named Bill Hatch, and asked if I would know a Bill Hatch. There were more than 500 million people in India and none that I knew was named Bill Hatch, but I thought one of my brothers might know him. Woman-like, I tried to keep the ball in play. He asked if I would mention it to my brothers, and then asked if I would mind his writing me. I gladly gave him my address and we corresponded after I left for medical school. By this time he had changed his mind about the ministry, deciding to go into medicine instead, and he entered the medical school at the University of Cincinnati. I never did get to meet Bill Hatch, or to hear about him again, but I did marry the man who asked about him. His name was Bill McGarey.

I finished medical school in Philadelphia while Bill finished his medical training in Cincinnati. I was able to get an internship at Deaconess Hospital in Cincinnati, where I could be close to Bill. I was the only woman doing an internship at Deaconess, and that should have stirred a warning buzz in my stomach. I soon found out why they didn't have any place for me to sleep when I was on patient call. So I took a blanket and pillow and slept on an x-ray table. There was no phone in the x-ray room and when I got a call, I had to run down the hall to answer it. At this point I couldn't help thinking of the little English girl back in India who had said, "Women aren't doctors. They're nurses."

Three months into the internship I became pregnant. I had problems with morning sickness and other early pregnancy symptoms. My troubles really began when I went on surgery service. The resident in charge had been a surgeon in the armed forces and he soon made it clear that I was expendable. He believed firmly in three things and he made all three abundantly clear: one, women didn't belong in medicine; two, pregnant women didn't belong in medicine; three, I didn't belong in medicine. Not at Deaconess Hospital. Therefore, it became important to him to get me out of medicine, and it became equally important to me that he *not* succeed.

He did everything he could to make life difficult for me, scheduling me for the earliest and longest surgeries. This meant that I had to be in the operating room by 7:30 A.M., and the surgeries would frequently last for five hours or longer. I couldn't get any breakfast before surgery because the cafeteria didn't open until eight, and there were no vending machines in the hospital. So I would go into the operating room without any food, feeling very weak and shaky, but determined not to give in.

Aching in body and mind, I turned to God for help as I had done in childhood. It arrived in the form of a little black angel named Lucille, an angel who posed as a maid working on the surgery floor. Nobody will ever tell me she wasn't an angel out of the blue. Without a word to anyone or from anyone, the posted surgery schedule began to miraculously change and my name was put down for nine o'clock surgery. This meant I could sleep later and still eat breakfast. My surgical resident accused me of changing the schedule, which I vehemently denied. And I would never have known about the guardian angel if I hadn't been in the hall on the way to a call at three o'clock one morning. I spotted her with a chair pulled up to the scheduling blackboard. She was erasing my name at the seven o'clock mark, substituting another intern's name and jotting my name down for nine o'clock. I gave thanks to this little guardian angel all the rest of my life. Had it not been for her, I would have lost the baby or become seriously ill. While I was no Joan of Arc or feminist activist, there was no way I was going to let this man push me out of medicine. I felt I had to do this not only for myself but for every woman who ever wanted to be a doctor. I believe this feeling helped me to carry on, this and the little black angel.

I made it through those early months of pregnancy working almost to the time our first child emerged, a lusty boy named Carl, destined to become a doctor himself one day. My husband was now in practice, and we were with him for the six months he worked in the back hills of Kentucky in conditions not unlike those I experienced in India. It was time well spent, when I was nursing my baby, being a housewife, and not practicing medicine. And it was time very dear and precious to me, as it took some doing to balance my obligations to my patients with those to my husband and a growing family.

Bill didn't have a missionary's call, so I arranged with the church to stay in this country. We became partners in family practice, first in the small town of Wellsville, Ohio, and then in Phoenix, Arizona, where we eventually established the A.R.E. Clinic. There we selectively combined the practice of conventional medicine with the uncanny wisdom of Edgar Cayce, the remarkable metaphysician known as the Sleeping Prophet. Growing up in India, I held a pragmatic, down-to-earth view about medicine. Bill felt the same way. Even if Cayce was right in his diagnoses about people he had never seen, and correct in the remedies he suggested, how could we as doctors adapt his comments to individual situations—and patients—about which he knew absolutely nothing? Cayce had died before we even began our practice.

Two areas of medicine particularly interested me: one was plastic surgery, the other, family practice. They were not that divergent. It wasn't the cosmetic phase of surgery that interested me, but the restructuring of faces horribly disfigured in accidents or in the horrors of war. I trained with a plastic surgeon for almost a year, but since Bill's primary interest was family practice, I visualized a partnership like that of my parents.

Bill had been reading everything he could find on Edgar Cayce, and he began looking into reincarnation. From my Indian watch this sounded like Hinduism. I thought, "Oh, my lord, he's become a Hindu." But the more I got into it, the more I realized that the concepts from the Edgar Cayce material were not really in opposition to my basic Christian beliefs. And coming from a deeply committed Christian background, I believed these concepts just added another dimension to what I already believed and was deeply committed to.

From Kentucky we went to Wellsville. The years in Wellsville were formative years for me as a physician. Wellsville was a small river town on the Ohio River. Most of the people worked in the nearby steel mills or in the local pottery and brickyards. When we started our practice, there were eight doctors. By the time Bill was called into service during the Korean war, there were just three doctors. One had a heart attack, the other was a refugee who could speak little English, and then there was me—with thousands of patients. All of the house calls fell on my shoulders. By this time we had four children, and I frequently took the two older children along with me. I enjoyed their company, but since there were many 24-hour days, I also had no choice. I thought of my mother and dad working in the jungle with the sick and I kept on going.

On top of everything else, there was also a mumps epidemic going on at the time. Our children got the mumps first, and then, in my fatigued state, I too got the mumps and almost died. A pregnant patient of mine, severely hemorrhaging, called me in desperation. I was running a fever but felt I had to go to her. She had no one else. I spent some time with her and when I finally got back home, I had an agonizing back pain, like nothing I'd ever experienced before. I had developed a mumps nephritis, an infection of the kidney. Mumps is tougher on grown-ups. A visiting physician friend came by and examined me. She shook her head and put me in the hospital, ordering complete rest and no visitors, not even my children. There was one problem. The hospital patients soon found out where I was and they would troop up the backstairs to seek my advice. So my life-saving physician and her husband took me into their home and nursed me through it, while my housekeeper stayed around the clock with the four kids. I'd talk to them on the phone, and after a few days they could visit. I finally returned home after passing a kidney stone.

I was ready to move on when Bill came out of the service. I rhapsodized about the wonderful dry, healthful climate and the sparkling environment of the Arizona desert country. I took the children with me and flew out to Arizona, a move I have never regretted. We opened a joint family practice which eventually became the A.R.E. Clinic. Bill had become an ardent believer in Cayce and by this time had fully explored reincarnation, a concept that the fundamentalist Cayce had turned up in the trance state where he usually visualized his healings and prophecies of world events.

In the beginning, though intrigued by its plausibility, I wasn't totally convinced, still clinging to the traditional Christian doctrine which excluded reincarnation as a viable belief. However, not wanting to close off my mind, I turned to the Bible, and found to my surprise several references to reincarnation, notably, when Jesus asked his disciples, "Whom do men say that I the Son of Man am?"

And the disciples replied, "Some say thou art John the Baptist. Some, Elijah, and others Jeremiah."

And Jesus replied, "I say unto you that Elijah is come already, and they knew him not, but have done unto him whatsoever they listed. Likewise shall also the Son of Man suffer of them."

They knew then that he was talking about John the Baptist. And as Bill said, "If they weren't talking about reincarnation, what were they talking about?"

Beyond this, and more in keeping with our identity as physicians, were the remarkable remedies of this strange man. Most notable was the cold-processed castor oil, known as the Palma Christi, the hand of Christ, which released intestinal obstructions and kidney stones when used as external packs. Cayce also talked about coordination between organs like the kidneys and liver, which, when imbalanced, could lead to serious illness. He seemed to have more of a rational grasp of body function than any medical source I was acquainted with. It was astounding, since he had no medical training and was getting all this in trance. If it worked, and could be replicated, I saw no reason not to use his remedies when proven by results to be effective and safe—very much the same standard that conventional medicine sets for itself.

Cayce saw the big picture. Essentially, he saw the mind, body and spirit as one, and each person as an entity and energy force distinct from everybody else. And in deference to this distinctness, Cayce's suggestions varied from person to person, though the disease or malfunction treated might be the same. For me, the psychic readings dealing with prayer, dream therapy and the body-mind connection were not difficult. I had watched my parents deal in these areas of consciousness all my life and I knew that medicine and healing had to be a total approach. I agreed with Cayce that the patient was more than the disease.

Bill and I had been examining the Cayce material for more than a year without having the slightest notion of how we could use it. It made no medical sense in light of our conventional medical training. Hugh Lynn Cayce, the head of the Cayce Foundation in Virginia Beach, dropped by while he was in Phoenix, and knowing of our interest, said, "Why don't you people do something with my father's physical readings?"

We shrugged and explained that even when it worked for Edgar Cayce it was all Greek to us because we couldn't psychically differentiate the treatment for the same ailment with each distinctive case as he had. "Your father was psychic, he understood when things needed to be changed. We are not psychics. We're down-to-earth doctors."

Eventually, as we really got into the Cayce material, we realized that behind every Cayce health reading there were broad psychological and physical concepts that made sense. He was not dealing with cookbook medicine, but with pragmatic concepts which had to do with how the body functions and how different internal systems had to coordinate to insure the well-being of the whole. He spoke about coordination between the liver and the spleen, something we had not heard of in medical school. He spoke about coordination between the sympathetic and parasympathetic systems—which we did know about. He went into lymphatic drainage, the body's way of keeping individual cells clean and healthy. This made good sense, and it made the effectiveness of cold-processed castor oil packs understandable if they stimulated this activity. As Cayce indicated, each cell in the body had an innate intelligence of its own, and sent out a message when it needed help. Cayce picked out that message. "It was almost," said Bill, "as if an injured ankle, swollen with the pain, had said, 'I'm hurt and need a little castor oil rubbed over me.'"

It wasn't that simple for us. But when these situations kept recurring, and a swollen ankle or elbow responded to the castor oil, or whatever Cayce suggested, then we had something substantial. It was important to us medically to understand the concept behind any Cayce remedy, just as if we were dealing with conventional medicine.

Oddly, the fact that Cayce had no conscious knowledge of what he was saying made an impression on me. There was no twisting of words, no wish to impress. As I saw how his recommendations invariably worked, I noticed that the treatment was innocuous, however it worked. I also learned that Cayce had sent hundreds of the ailing to therapist Harold Reilly's Health Center in New York, without being consciously aware of Reilly's name. Reilly spoke of these cases freely. All had benefited from treatments jotted down on pieces of paper. Obviously, we were not dealing with an ordinary man.

Cayce's philosophy was as unusual as his health readings. Believing in a continuity of life, he considered our life on this planet to be a testing ground. I learned soon enough how this test could turn a person's life around.

Bill and I appeared to have the ideal partnership. We had six children and a thriving clinic that attracted patients and medical observers from all over the world. We lectured together, traveled together and enjoyed our family life together. At 70, after 46 years of marriage, there didn't seem to be a dark spot on the horizon. And then out of the blue my physician husband came to me and asked for a divorce. He wanted to marry another woman. I looked at him in dismay and disbelief. We had not only shared a strong family life, we were also almost lifelong partners in the practice of medicine which we loved and worked at so well together. Our world-renowned clinic, using various disciplines of medicine, had helped us to grow in thought and action, grateful that we could help patients who so often came to us as a last resort.

And now it had all ended in the flash of a few spoken words. My life was in disarray. My husband kept the clinic we had founded. I wished him and his new wife well. It would have been alien to my nature to have done otherwise. But now, at 70, beyond the pale in most professions, how was I to begin a new life? I had my dreary moments. I had no money. I drove around in an old battered car. I didn't even have an office in which to hang my hat or my shingle. But I did have something I could never lose: the memories of my life in the outbacks of India and a stern-visaged father with a kindly eye who said, "You never quit. Never, never, never. You've lost nothing until you quit. Whether it's a footrace or the game of life."

Nothing could change the wonderful memories Bill and I shared, but I knew I had to go on. I set about to rebuild my life. I was amazed by the number of friends and patients who implored me to go on with my practice. Some said with tears in their eyes, "How can you leave us?" The irony was not lost on me. I was able to laugh when I thought I would never laugh again. In that moment I saw the road ahead and it was straight and clear. The God I worshipped in childhood had never left me. I could hear my mother's voice resonating in my ears. "Listen to what is in your heart and you will find him."

My six children rallied to my support. There wasn't anything they wouldn't have done for me. And my youngest daughter, Helene, who had been associated with me in family practice, together with her husband Fred, a psychologist, joined me in planning a new clinic.

I thought of the patients so dear to me. I remembered what I had told so many about standing tall and taking hold of their own life—all the things my mother and dad had instilled in us when we were growing up. Yes, growing up. Fighting to survive myself, I thought of the special breed of patients I knew as "the survivors." I thought of Grace Page, in her 80s, who had lost her husband and had about every sickness there was. Yet she came to work in my office every day with a smile on her face and a will to help the sick. I thought of the 90-year-old martinet with a cancer mass on her chest who said it was no problem, she'd get the best of it. And she did. And then there was the younger woman, divorced by a doctor, who used me as a role model to end her drinking after a hard divorce and the death of two sons. Yes, I owed them all something. I had meant something to them. They were my partners in healing. And they had kept me going all these years. I wasn't finished. I wasn't about to end our partnership now. That's what partnerships were all about. Like Mother and Dad. Until death do us part. And then some. I had my partners, my children, my friends. And my heritage. And the energy and vitality of a younger woman, willed to me by parents who served well into their 90s. And who still live in my heart.

I have my own clinic now, and people in need who come to me for help. I feel needed. And I have made a great discovery. I found that a doctor can often heal herself in helping others to heal themselves.

Stella: The Human Will Is Supreme

*Each patient carries
his own doctor inside him.
They come to us not knowing that
truth. We are at our best when
we give the doctor who resides
in each patient a chance
to go to work.*

—Dr. Albert Schweitzer

She had struck me as the picture of youth and beauty when she was young. And with time, the elegance and charm, the childlike good looks, still clung to her. The eyes were sparkling, the symmetrical face was unlined, the thick dark hair crowned her beauty.

Now she was dying in a New York hospital and the nation's heart went out to her. There was nothing more her doctors could do for her but send her home to die. All they had had was chemotherapy and radiation. The chemotherapy had taken what strength the cancer had left, and had lined the face that time couldn't touch.

She had not lived long after that, and the nation mourned the passing of Jacqueline Kennedy, whose life had been an emblem of grace and courage.

Two thousand miles to the west, in Scottsdale, Arizona, a woman of about the same age, afflicted with the same dread disease—cancer of the lymph glands, lymphoma—was staging a heroic recovery. She, too, had been in a New York hospital, not only for the lymphoma but for an advanced case of gangrene. Doctors had already taken part of one leg, and planned to take the other leg. "Have your husband order you a wheelchair," they said. She looked at them. They had already told her that chemotherapy was her only hope, and now they were telling her she would never walk again. But she was a fighter. She looked deep into herself and remembered how she had come out to Arizona four years before and cured her "incurable asthma" when nobody else could. She phoned me now, as she had then, and I said, "Come along and we'll see how we can help you help yourself."

The patient, Stella Andres, never saw herself as a victim. She came out to Scottsdale with her husband and they took a house. She had seen how people had suffered with chemotherapy, losing their vitality and strength, sometimes becoming only shadows of themselves, and then losing their will to live. She had decided it was not going to happen to her. She was not going to lose her hair, the mark of her womanhood, nor her wits, the gift of her Greek ancestry.

She had arrived with her husband George, a stalwart support. That was important. She needed to feel she was not alone. She needed to feel she could beat the cancer and the gangrene, just as she had beaten back the asthma that was once choking the life out of her. As I examined her I noted not only the swollen nodes that were the signs of her cancer, but the spark in her eye and the set of her jaw. She was an older woman, 60 or so, but not old. Life was just as sweet to her at this time as it was in her youth. She had much to live·for—a family, things she wanted to do and people she wanted to help.

She had two ailments to consider: the cancer, of course, which sometimes responded to conventional treatment, and the gangrene, which almost never did. But she had learned a lot from her earlier healing and knew it was not the disease she had to work with but herself. She had to summon up the same attitude, the same mind power, the same tenaciousness that had helped her four years earlier. I smiled as I looked at her. There was no sign of defeat in her face, no doubts or misgivings. She looked on me as her partner—someone treating the whole person and not the symptoms—in this, the greatest battle of her life.

Stella knew what she had to do from the start—adopt a mindset that brooked no failure. "You know what the first steps are?" I said.

She nodded. "Yes, get rid of the negativity inside and around me, the long faces that reflect thoughts of dying. I must think of living on and the things I want to do: the morning sunshine and the lush green fields, the hills of home, the evening stars, a baby's smile, the people I love. And the God I believe in, the overseer of my universe. Yes, my universe, for I belong here. I must think of Jesus, the greatest of healers, and of the angels, who stood at the foot of my bed once before and smiled. They didn't speak. The love in their faces said it all: 'Have faith. You will be well.' I never doubted. They were just as I saw them as a child, always serene, with a white aura, a look of peace."

Stella had her dreams as well. They came in tandem with her visions. She didn't speak of them, not at the time, but she kept a dream journal on her night table. The dreams came out of a subconscious mind so often prophetic and revealing. In one dream she saw herself walking on water. It brought a smile to her face. It could signify only one thing: a miracle. Nearing the shore she saw a fisherman haul in a fish. She felt buoyed and uplifted.

The visions, too, were very real to Stella. The archangel Michael, the most constant of the angels, stood tall and erect. She felt his strength pouring through her veins. At the low point of her illness, in the New York hospital, the doctors gave her a year or two without chemotherapy. And they gave up on her gangrenous leg. They had already cut her three times, amputating the other leg. She thought of her angels and the will within her. She cried, "You're not taking my one good leg." With that she took over, and was still taking over, sharing her recovery with me.

Getting out of the hospital in New York was like getting a charge of electricity for Stella. At the Scottsdale Holistic Medical Group in Arizona, the staff threw their arms around her and kissed her, just as they had when she had her "incurable" asthma. So it was like coming home. She had done it before with her asthma, through nutrition, exercise, visualization and the spirit within. And now we were going to do it again with the lymphoma and the gangrene. She was put on a strict regimen of diet, exercise and cold-processed castor oil packs— some of which she had gone through with the asthma that had choked off her lungs. The mind and spirit, stirring within her body, animated her immune system, and the dreams of walking on water sent her a message. She laughed as she told me about it. "After walking on water I figured I could do almost anything. Getting well will be a breeze."

And it was. In six months Stella tested negative for the lymphoma and the toes on her good leg had resumed their normal tone and color. The doctors at St. Vincent's in New York were awed. They'd heard of "spontaneous" cancer remissions without really believing in them. But gangrene? This was a first.

Stella's treatment was unconventional but inclusive, incorporating aspects of holistic, allopathic and homeopathic medicine. We even had her soaking her gangrenous toes in the detergent Biz for 20 minutes twice a day, to help her shed the black skin from her toes. The Biz people might have been surprised about that, perhaps not realizing that the enzyme in their product had such therapeutic value.

After this cure, everybody at the clinic congratulated Stella on being out of a wheelchair and walking. She didn't even use a cane after a while. One day, she marched triumphantly into my office. When I looked up and said nothing about her walking, she couldn't help but say, "Dr. Gladys, didn't you notice I'm walking?"

I smiled. "Stella, I've never thought of you as not walking."

After that, Stella became something of an evangelist for holistic medicine and the human spirit. She and her husband, a retired businessman, had taken a home in Chandler, a Scottsdale-Phoenix suburb, and Stella became involved with therapy support groups, freely giving counsel on how she beat the cancer. "If I can do it, you can do it," she would often say to another patient. And she frequently quoted me, saying as I so often did, "Always remember, the human will is supreme." Or she repeated the mystic Cayce's wise words: "The spirit and mind are the builders. The physical is the result."

Stella had herself checked up at the clinic periodically, and her regimen worked for 11 years. She remained cancer-free. One day she came into my Scottsdale clinic for a routine physical. As I was going over her as usual, my hands stopped at a solid mass over Stella's abdomen and then retraced their movements. Something was radically wrong. Tests followed. They only confirmed what I already thought: The lymphoma was back.

We looked at each other and I liked what I saw. As before, there was no fear in her eyes, only a reflective look as if she were wondering how it had happened.

I smiled and gave her an embrace. "We did it once before," I said. "We can do it again. You are living proof of that."

Stella had become a miracle woman in the eyes of many people. They wondered how she had done it, and her story had grown with the telling. She was a living legend. She had visualized the gangrene away with an imaginary swordfish shearing away the odious black skin with their swords. She had little dogs nibbling away at the lymphatic nodes that recorded her cancer. With a prosthesis fitted to one leg, and the leg she had saved, she walked and drove a car as ably as she ever had.

Now the bubble of invincibility had burst. Where were those angels? Where were Jesus and the archangel Michael? And what of me, her partner? All this time, Stella had visualized me sitting at her bedside, healing her body, holding her hand. Her visualizations were so powerful, they reached deep into her subconscious mind, directing healing alpha brain waves to any area of the body she chose.

Now here she was, a decade later, in her 60s, like Jacqueline Kennedy, compelled to take on this adversary again. How had it happened? She asked that question of herself a dozen times. Then she brushed this thought aside and looked deep inside herself, with the same subconscious mind that had beaten the lymphoma so long ago. She had almost forgotten it was there for her.

Forgotten. The word lingered. Was this the key? Had she lost the humility that had always characterized everything she did? Had she begun to think herself superior to the sick who didn't have the same discipline she had? She stuck to a stringent diet of fruits and vegetables, maintained a rigid exercise routine and meditated for hours on end on the lymphatic nodes that covered her body. Painstakingly, she had applied castor oil packs over the liver area to stimulate the immune system and assist in the detoxifying process. And she had continued with the periodic colonics she had found so embarrassing and demeaning in the beginning.

She never played doctor, but she gave the people who came to her certain guidelines that anyone who had beaten cancer might pass on to a friend.

"No fats, no sugar, no meat," she'd say, and see the horror in some eyes. No meat? "It was like they would die if they had to forgo meat or sweets." She stressed a strictly vegetarian diet in the beginning, a purifying diet, and she got impatient at times when people couldn't conform. "I should have followed Dr. Gladys's example. She never got impatient with anyone. She never lost faith. 'Just do the best you can,' she'd say, and she'd give a patient a little hug or a pat on the back."

I thought about what Stella had said. I questioned that a loss of humility would lead so quickly to a loss of grace. Stella was hardly a sinner. Hadn't Peter asked the Master, "How oft shall I forgive? Till seven times?" And hadn't Jesus replied, "Not until seven times. But until 70 times seven. And more if necessary."

No, it had to be something else. I had taken care of Stella periodically for 11 years, and when the diagnosis of the recurrence of her lymphoma was confirmed, we decided that if she had beaten it before, she could do it again. We would work together at it, using both holistic and conventional medicine. Stella went to see a local oncologist who had worked with her before and had been supportive. And she continued her work at our clinic.

We began again with the visualization and the diet. She had pretty much stopped the special diet, and she now became acutely aware that she needed to continue with it. She also was not doing any active visualization. Life moved on, she became very busy, and she both felt and behaved like a well person. And she was, up to a point.

It was easy to understand, and quite human, Stella's wanting to return to a normal routine when free of an illness for so long. There were no excesses on her part: no alcohol, no smoking. But lymphoma does have a way of returning. So we resumed the healing.

The previous time, when Stella would get low on protein, we would add fish to her diet. This appeared to help and she returned to a regular diet. When she got sick again, after 11 years, we put her back on a fruit and vegetable diet. After a while we added more protein—fish—to maintain her strength. She had been very active, feeling it was her mission to let people know that they could heal themselves like she had. She may have been doing too much, depleting her energy. The lymphatic nodes were again putting pressure on the large blood vessels and affecting her circulation. She also had a longtime heart problem which was now acting up, and her cardiologist wasn't upbeat about her prognosis. He told her he was not at all sure her heart would hold up for more than a year without cardiac surgery. But Stella still had a lot going for her, and her indomitable spirit. She reminded me of what I had said about the human will being supreme. Even with her arrhythmia, and a heart valve problem she rarely mentioned, Stella had no doubt she was going to make it. She had faith in her angels and felt that they wouldn't let her down, not after all the comfort they had given her before.

We decided on another cardiologist, one who would be supportive. Stella began to improve, but then she had a flu which affected her lungs. Everything seemed to be going against her now. She broke a blood vessel and had a huge hematoma, a hemorrhage under her skin. The loss of blood pulled her down. She had trouble visualizing because of her bleeding and her breathing difficulty. She got so bad that they rushed her to the nearest hospital. It was like her whole system had shut down. But that night she again rallied. I saw the light in her eyes and I knew then that she would be all right.

I decided I could leave for India as I had planned for some time, but I remained with Stella in her consciousness. She visualized my sitting there by the bedside, holding her hand, and all the time I was away I was praying for her. She saw that as well. It was probably more effective than had I been there bodily, for she used me to symbolize the doctor within her, reaching into her highest level of consciousness, the healing alpha level.

My daughter Helene attended Stella while I was away, and when I got back, she was on the mend. There had been talk of chemotherapy, but Stella had rejected it as before.

A renewed Stella was barely out of the hospital when she met up with a reporter skeptical of her miraculous recovery. She had been through a succession of illnesses that would have finished off the average person, yet I saw nothing of her ordeal in her face or voice. She stood erect, with poise, and gave the reporter a firm handshake. She had a classical face, handsome and surprisingly youthful.

"They tell me you're a walking miracle," the reporter began.

"I don't give myself that much credit." Stella spoke matter-of-factly as they sat across from each other. She had driven to their appointment.

She gave him a piercing look, then folded her hands on the desk in front of her and said with a smile, "Well?"

He smiled back, sizing her up.

"What was your reaction when the cancer came back?"

"I was annoyed."

"Annoyed?"

"Yes, disgusted. I should have kept a closer watch on my regimen. Stayed longer with my angels." She laughed under her breath.

His eyebrows went up. "Angels?"

"I see angels when I think of my father. He had so much to do with whatever spirituality I have. He passed away shortly before I came out to Arizona. He was a Greek immigrant with an inquiring mind. He used to talk to me about Nostradamus and the Greek philosopher Plato and the ancient prophets when I was a teenager. It embarrassed me in front of my friends—you know how young people are—and so he stopped talking to me about things metaphysical until he lay sick and dying years later in a nursing home. I spent every day with him. I had read about Edgar Cayce by this time and I was interested in the spiritual."

The reporter frowned. "And how does all this figure into your recovery?"

"I had a feeling of my connection to the universe. I drew strength from it. I was part of it all. My father talked to me about the stars and the moon and the tides and the effect they had on our minds and bodies. He talked to me about the prophets and Jesus, with his special connection to the Lord. He made it clear to me that all these figures, especially Jesus and the angels, still lived on in the influence they had on our lives."

She looked away for a moment. There was a mist in her eyes, but she went on. "My father died when he finished what he had to teach me. I felt him with me that night in the hospital when I lost so much blood they thought I would die. Later that night I rallied. One doctor at the hospital said later that nobody as sick as I was had ever walked out of that hospital, but I knew I would. I could see Dr. Gladys in India, and what she was wearing. I saw Jesus and the angels. They hadn't left me. And I saw my father. He was smiling, and I knew what that meant. He wasn't ready for me yet."

The reporter wasn't that sure about angels. He had seen them as a boy, kneeling at his bed, but they disappeared as he grew older.

"So what will it be now?" the reporter asked.

Stella's eyes lit up.

"After coming home from the hospital I meditated, and in my meditation I asked to be guided. In my visualization, I saw Jesus and the angels as well as Mary and the archangel Michael. This is what I see when I meditate and visualize—that I am getting healing from Jesus, Mary, the archangel Michael. Jesus surrounds me in a white light, and my angels appear when I need them, in luminous white linen. They don't say anything, they don't have to. Their presence is enough.

"Through my experiences I have learned patience and humility. I thank God every day for giving me the time and strength to help others and to give them hope and inspiration. I stand before God with great humility and thank him for helping me see that each person is different and needs to heal in his or her own way. I stand beside them, encouraging them and helping them to do what they believe in. I hope to serve as a source of inspiration and to help in God's work the best way I know how. I want to be there for those who need me—to listen, to make suggestions and to allow them to come to me whenever they want.

"I wept when a gallant Jacqueline Kennedy fought for life and then succumbed to cancer after the same treatment that I had spurned.

"I knew what she must have gone through—the pain and despair, then the feeling of hopelessness as her strength waned. I thought of writing to her, but I had a feeling, with the chemotherapy and all, that she had made up her mind that it was time to move on. She left the hospital to be at home with her loved ones when the end came. She was a great lady. She is at peace now."

A shadow fell over Stella's face. "Of course what helped me might not have helped her. It is hard to say. We are all so different."

"But the will to live, isn't that the same?"

"In the beginning perhaps, but it must be nourished and encouraged by a doctor who is supportive and ready to share your healing. That is what I found in Dr. Gladys McGarey—a true partner in my time of need."

Have Hope

*T*he spirit and mind
are the builders, the body
the result.

—EDGAR CAYCE

I could see the new patient was uneasy. He looked past me instead of meeting my eye. He was middle-aged, stocky, well-dressed, with no perceivable illness. His eyes darted around the treatment room and passed over the credentials on my wall.

"Yes," I smiled, "I'm an M.D., twice an M.D., in fact."

"It's my first visit to a woman doctor," he said, almost apologetically. "I've been everywhere else."

I held back my smile. "I don't have any men patients or women patients. I only have patients. And many are children."

"My wife calls you the doctor of last resort."

I laughed and gave the patient a gentle pat on the shoulder. "We are all family here. When you walked through that door you became my family."

He looked at me. "That's a new one on me. Usually, I'm shuttled in and out, before I have a chance to say anything."

I could see the uneasiness and tension slip away, and I waited. I wanted him to talk about himself when he was ready. He looked up in surprise. The other doctors had always started the conversation off.

"I don't know what it is," he said finally. "I've been to a couple of doctors. They were no help. I ache all over, have no energy. I can't get going in the morning or sleep at night. They say it's psychosomatic."

He was a businessman, fairly successful, at an age when the dreams of youth had slipped away and the realities of life were dimming his expectations. Basically, there was nothing wrong with him that couldn't be cured with a little tender care. I made a mental note to call his wife. The worst thing for any patient is to feel abandoned. To be healed they need to feel secure and relaxed.

I recommended brisk outdoor walking and therapeutic body massage.

He had a surprised look. "No medicine?"

"No medicine. You're a healthy man." I thought of Hippocrates, the Father of Medicine, and his message for all doctors: "Thou shalt do no harm."

I allow patients to share in their healing. I delve deeply into their consciousness with them, knowing that the mind and the spirit are the builders, and the physical the result. And I listen. That's all-important.

Patients are the sum of everything they think and do, of their past and present, and their future hopes. A patient is not just a disease or a disability. A patient is a storehouse of significant memories waiting to be extracted in dreams and meditations which stir the soul and send it into action against any predator that threatens the body.

Patients come to me knowing only that I may have helped other people, and they don't really know or care how this was accomplished. Used to conventional medicine, they often sit back in astonishment as I talk about their aspirations and their dreams—the dreams of sleep—and meditations of such depth that they invoke the alpha brain waves that send healing messages to every cell of the body.

I am not a dream doctor. I will use whatever drugs, diet or exercise indicated in any health situation. But the best way we have of convincing a patient of the correctness of any therapy, however odd it may seem, is to heal him with that therapy.

I vividly recall the middle-aged skeptic I advised to dream his pain away. He'd had this pain in his chest for years and nobody could do anything for him, not even diagnose what it was. He tested negative for everything. This should have relieved him, but it didn't. He had an idea that all the doctors were thinking it was just in his head. But he knew it was in his chest—the pain was severe and distracting.

I believed him. I invariably believe the patient. What better source do I have? He also didn't want to hear that it was something he'd have to live with. I'm sure he'd heard that all too often. I gave him a thorough examination and came up empty like the other doctors had. It was an unusual case and unusual cases call for unusual approaches. I mulled over a thought that had come to me. I didn't want to drive him away, and I was convinced he had a very real problem—with his chest, not his head.

As all this was going on in my mind, the patient was looking around the room as if wondering what he was doing there. I had nothing else, so I asked him if he dreamed. He shook his head. "Everybody dreams," I said, "they just don't remember."

He frowned but a look of interest came to his eyes. I had hoped to pique his curiosity, and that was good enough for starters.

"I want you to keep a pencil and pad on your night table," I said. "Tell yourself just before bedtime that you're going to dream and you will remember whatever dream you have. It may take a few nights but it will happen."

His eyebrows went up, and I said, "It's worked for a good many people. I think it will work for you."

He shrugged and left. A week or so later he came back in a pensive sort of mood.

"Well?" I said.

He nodded a little sheepishly, "I don't know what to make of it. It was very strange. But it seemed real as I was dreaming it. It went back hundreds of years to the Crusades. I was a Crusader, dressed in mail like the rest of the soldiers, with the insignia of the Cross." He stopped suddenly to see how I was reacting and saw I was listening. He went on. "I was charging forward with the others on some sort of installation—like a fort. We were meeting considerable resistance when a spear flung by one of the defenders pierced my armor and went into my chest."

I could see a look of pain in his eyes, as though he were reliving it all again. And he was, in his own very human way.

I could almost see it happening. It had been a gaping wound, a mortal wound, and the trauma of the moment remained—all the anger, hate and frustration—locked in the innate intelligence of every cell. It was very real in his consciousness or it wouldn't have materialized in the dream. I told him he'd have to forgive and forget, then forgive himself for the grievance he bore so close to his heart.

He looked at me, then nodded. The physician within would take it from there.

The possibilities were intriguing: reincarnation perhaps, or the humanist Jung's concept of racial consciousness, remembrances of body and mind passed through the genes of countless generations. We see it in animals. You throw a puppy in the water and he'll swim. He doesn't have to be taught. We know of dogs who go into a corner or under a bed to mourn a master who has died at that same moment, but hundreds of miles away. Likewise, deep inside the patient there's a storehouse of memories manifested in dreams, meditations and the vague stirrings of the soul.

I feel it's important to think both like a patient and like a physician. It's the indispensable ingredient of any great doctor— a caring nature that looks deep into the human heart, mind and spirit. All join together in the fight for life. The body is never helpless. Its immune system, awakened, is capable of staving off any disease. The body contains genes which have lived before, which have overcome plagues and other disasters. Those cells have an awareness sufficient to quell any invader if they are not stifled by fear and indifference.

I believe strongly not only in wellness but in wholeness, and in the whole person: body, mind and spirit. This respect for the whole person even extends to those people for whom medicine can no longer help. They can be shown how to leave this life with a feeling of hope and accomplishment, looking beyond to a new world.

How people live determines how they die. In both, they can be courageous and resolute, believing in something greater than themselves—God, Jesus, or whatever animates the spirit of love and life within. This is very much the task of the physician within, who is both doctor and patient, and who leads the assault on the intruder feeding on one's body and mind.

There is no wellness unless the whole body is functioning at its peak. The weak organ soon spreads its weakness to other parts of the body which must then work harder to maintain a healthy body and outlook—what I call wholeness. This is the reason for holistic medicine, which calls on any therapy of established worth to help the patient heal himself.

As one of the cofounders of the American Holistic Medical Association, I also serve on the National Institutes of Health Committee that determines research guidelines for alternative medicine. Since I became a physician, I have worked to join alternative medicine with the conventional and the traditional. At our clinic, where we combine the best of alternative and traditional medicine, disease is a transient visitor. There is a relaxed air, a friendly ambiance, from therapeutic massage to soothing music, special exercises, detoxifying diets and always humor. Mostly we strive to get patients to understand their illness, so they can participate in the cure.

I'm never too busy to sit down and talk with a patient. They tell me more than they realize and I seldom cut them off. They are my teachers as well as my patients. They are my friends. Not all doctors take the same view.

I also listen to doctors as well as patients, especially doctors who gripe about patients.

"Can you imagine," said a doctor friend, "this patient coming into my office and telling me what's wrong with her? She goes on about her aches and pains, then tells me she thinks she's got appendicitis. I never heard anything so absurd, her making her own diagnosis."

This doctor didn't know—or care—about the physician within and she angrily cut the patient off. "Where did you get your medical degree?" she asked the patient.

The patient shrank into her chair. "I'm sorry," she responded, her eyes lowered.

"They talk," the physician went on, "like they have a degree from Johns Hopkins."

I mulled this over. "By the way," I said, "where do you think Jesus got his medical degree?"

Two women had a strong impact on the direction I took. My mother, Beth Taylor, and my Aunt Belle, both of whom cared for the sick that nobody else seemed to care about. The mystique and lore of the East are in my blood. My father, a staunch Presbyterian, was driven by the lure of a land—India—that seemed to loom out of a distant past. My brother, Gordon Taylor, a minister, carries on the tradition, ministering to 600 Indian children of leper parents. Many of these children go on to become physicians and nurses.

When I visited India some years ago, my Aunt Belle was in her late 80s, caring for 130 children of leper parents. Her spirit was undaunted. I saw that she was building a cow shed and asked if she had a cow. "No, but if I build the shed, God will provide the cow." And he did. When Aunt Belle died at 94, she had over 200 children in her care, and several cows.

My mother also died in her 90s, after a bad fall. I remember helping my father lift her off a gurney onto an x-ray table. I'll never forget how she looked up at us, saw the pain in our faces and said with a smile, "The old gray mare, she ain't what she used to be."

I watched my mother cling to life, holding on by virtue of the bond with my dad. But she who had healed so many knew it was time for her to go. It was Good Friday, the day their great healer went to the cross to show that life was everlasting. She was ready too. She turned to my father, seeing the mist in his eyes and said, "John, you should have your lunch now."

He knew what she meant. Shortly after he left the hospital room, her spirit, joined so long to his, was able to move on. She died with a smile on her face.

My mother was laid to rest three days later, during the cele-
bration of the Resurrection. At the services I looked up in the
heavens and saw two rainbows arched across the sky. It was
something I would never forget and would carry in my heart
always. Mother's gentleness and humor in the face of death was
a great solace to me over the course of many hours dealing with
dying and death as I cared for patients.

I made several visits to the Far East. I enjoy traveling when I
can, and it can be instructive. During one trip to China early on,
I learned about the ancient art of acupuncture and how to join
conventional allopathic medicine with the homeopathic, and
also bring meditation into the treatment room. During another
trip, I joined up with my brother, Dr. Carl Taylor, a former head
of the United Nations International Children's Emergency Fund
in China, and of the Department of International Health
Medicine at Johns Hopkins Medical Center. I visited China and
Tibet with a medical research mission he headed that was spon-
sored by the two governments and Johns Hopkins.

Our trip took us to one of the women's and children's hospitals built when my brother headed UNICEF. One doctor's face
lit up when she recognized my brother. "Every woman and
child in Tibet has better health because of you," she said. She
addressed me as "the professor's little sister."

I assisted with the natal and maternal health services while I
was there. The deliveries were simple. There were no midwives
so the mothers usually delivered the babies themselves. I was
pleased to hear the mothers say that their husbands helped.
"How?" I asked a mother.

"He held the candle," the mother replied.

They still cut the umbilical cord with any instrument that was
handy—rusty scissors, knives, whatever was available—and tied
the cord with old wool. Then the baby was immediately swad-
dled, wrapped in rags, its arms bound to its sides. Knowing that

this binding process contributed to many pneumonia cases and deaths among newborns, I stressed the importance of the infants' being able to move their arms while crying, and thus expand their lungs. The mothers smiled gratefully and nodded.

I have seen medicine evolve over the years. Once novel ideas in healing are now casually accepted: eating fresh vegetables and fruits every day; warding off cancer of the colon by consuming roughage and whole grain foods; using acupuncture for pain, arthritis and asthma. Early on, when some of us counseled having fathers in the delivery room, this was considered an unsettling and even dangerous idea. Now it is common practice. Under fire, I sometimes questioned my own convictions, but I saw new alternative methods working and patients profiting, and I applauded the increasing attention paid to combining the holistic approach with the allopathic in treating trauma, bacterial infections, and medical and surgical emergencies.

Run-ins with the medical establishment were to be expected. I didn't listen to the pharmaceutical industry's twaddle; I didn't pass out antibiotics or sleeping pills like they were candy drops, though I prescribed drugs whenever I thought them necessary. And often I heard myself described as a witch doctor because I used remedies from Edgar Cayce, the Sleeping Prophet who diagnosed illnesses in his sleep and prescribed remedies, often with obscure herbs, that healed people. Cayce had often cured the lame, given the mortally ill a new lease on life and eased a variety of aches and pains. Whatever gift he had he attributed to his faith in God and Christ. Yet critics who had never healed anyone called him an anti-Christ.

Coming from a land where the belief in reincarnation was almost universal, I was drawn to Cayce by his references to past lives and their influence on the present. As I pored over the readings he had left behind, I was intrigued by the cures reported by the desperately ill who had asked for these psychic healings from him. I checked them out, and I checked on the doctors involved.

My study of the Edgar Cayce information broadened my horizons. I didn't want to get stuck only in what we learned in medical school. My job was helping people. Cayce also helped the sick who came to him, and if his methods worked for patients with symptoms similar to those I was seeing, then they had proved themselves. Yet people who knew nothing of Cayce said we were doing the work of the devil. They were the same kind of people who ridiculed Louis Pasteur when he discovered an invisible predator we all know today: bacteria.

Cayce was a fundamentalist Christian, but he was different from many of the fundamentalists we hear of today because he practiced his religion. What made him more of a target was his belief in reincarnation and the continuity of life.

My adversaries in the medical establishment were concerned about by my reputation for healing patients that other doctors had found "incurable," and their wrath extended to my children—three of whom had applied to the University of Arizona medical school. Carl, now an orthopedic surgeon in Houston, was the first to be turned down by the school's admitting board. Helene, now with me in the Scottsdale Holistic Medical Group, got the same treatment. David, the youngest, was also rejected, but he asked the committee why he didn't qualify. There was some hemming and hawing. In the end, the committee said, in effect, "Because your name is McGarey."

My children went on to other medical schools and none of us harbors the slightest resentment. In the end, I thought it a blessing because they ended up training in an open environment where new ideas could take root and flourish.

My difficulties with the "good old boys" in the medical establishment were ongoing. As a homeopathic doctor, as well as an allopath, I was chairman of the Arizona Homeopathic Board of

Medical Examiners. Nevertheless, I was hauled before a hostile allopathic Arizona Board of Medical Examiners, and charged, among other things, with not accepting normal standards of medicine. I responded and brought a lawyer. Before me I saw a tribunal of hostile doctors sitting in judgment with relentless eyes. All but a handful were male and I saw little encouragement there. The question wasn't even whether I was practicing witchcraft, but what *kind* of witchcraft. Even my lawyer blinked at the thought of a sleeping prophet, who had never gotten out of grade school, healing people he had never seen. It was conveniently overlooked that I was traditionally trained as well, and had a wider background than any of my accusers.

It hadn't occurred to any of my judges that they were prosecuting a chairman of another Arizona medical board—the Homeopathic Board of Medical Examiners—on the same level as their allopathic board, with a different approach. Homeopathy administers minute doses of a remedy designed to attack an illness by recreating the same symptoms in the patient. Homeopathic doctors were state-licensed, qualified medical doctors with the same privileges as allopaths. Why would any board of medical examiners challenge another Arizona state medical examiner?

It didn't look good for me, but I held on to my composure. Only the morning before, I had had a dream I found reassuring. Before retiring I had meditated and said a prayer, then fell off to sleep. In my dream, which I recalled in the morning, I was in my kitchen with the comedian Bob Hope, who was doing the dishes with me. He was saying it was his job to make people laugh. "And sometimes things I say are not particularly funny but people laugh anyway." I put my arm around him and said comfortingly that it was all right. "We all have things to do that we don't quite understand."

It was on the surface a silly sort of dream, but as I examined it from my dream experience, the word "hope" stood out. Still,

I saw little to laugh about. Everything was going the wrong way. I saw it in so many of the doctors' faces as one after another pecked away at me. I sighed to myself and looked at my lawyer. My medical license was on the table and we both knew it. One doctor in particular was out to get me, roundly denouncing me from his judgment seat. I was a disgrace to a noble profession.

The chairman of the board was sifting through his papers. He seemed preoccupied for a moment and then raised his hand to get the attention of the board. He had made a discovery and now he was about to share it, getting the attention of the board. He had come to a conclusion—belatedly, but still a conclusion: The attack on the therapeutic modalities of Dr. McGarey concerned holistic remedies, outside the jurisdiction of the allopathic medical board, despite McGarey's allopathic ties. The case was closed.

A long silence ensued. The one pesky doctor tried to continue his assault, but the chairman waved him down. "The meeting is over. If you want to talk to her, talk to her in the hall."

I found him waiting for me. He was unable to contain his anger. He pushed his face close to mine and growled, "Now let me tell you something, honey."

I was no feminist, and I had no difficulty competing with men. But this was all too much for me. I exploded. I began pounding on the man's shoulder with a heavy six-inch long metal key chain. "Don't you dare call me 'honey!' I am your peer, age-wise and professionally. And you will not call me 'honey.'"

He blushed, stammered and retreated into the meeting room. I heard waves of laughter. My lawyer, standing at the door, was holding his sides. I joined in. This, I realized, was what my "hope" dream was all about. Have hope and laugh your troubles away. I have been doing just that for some 50 years as a physician—homeopathic and allopathic.

A Divine Order

Physician, heal thyself.

—LUKE 4:23

My son, who is now a very good orthopedic surgeon, came to me when he had just finished his internship and said, "Mom, I'm worried. Here I am with all this training, and I'm going to go out and work with people who are depending on me. I'll have people's lives in my hands. It scares me. I don't know if I can handle it."

Having struggled with this same problem myself, I was able to answer him. "Carl, as a surgeon you may pull an incision together and suture it well, but you cannot make it heal. If you think you are the one who does the healing, you have a right to be scared. But if you understand that you are a channel through which healing moves, and that you are contacting the healing force within your patients, you have nothing to fear. You will have awakened the physician within them and sent them on their way to cure themselves."

I explained that it was our job to give the patient the will and purpose to go on, to do more and be better, to love and be loved, to visit with God every once in a while. We use every form of medicine—alternative and conventional—that works. We bring the patient into the fight and we bring ourselves into the fight. We share. It is a partnership.

We work with people by helping them to make the choices that will bring about their healing. But in the end, the will of the person is supreme—nothing is stronger than the human will fortified by faith.

All of us too often forget our connection with the universe. We have to tell ourselves that we're boundless, limitless and infinite—in an infinite world. We can do anything we want to do if we want it enough. When people used to ask me who I was, I'd say, "Dr. Gladys McGarey, and I am a physician." Then one day I thought, you know, that's wrong. I am Gladys McGarey, and I work as a physician. If I think I'm just a physician, that's all I am. But if I'm a person who works as a physician, then I can do a lot of other things. It was a liberating thought to me.

Likewise, when we identify with diseases, we can forget who we really are and that we are all unique. If a person says, "I have cancer," or "I am a cancer victim," or "I am an MS patient," or "I have lupus," that's what they become. To get away from this view can be very difficult. Affirmations are essential to changing our perspective. We need to say: "I am my own person. I am the master of my fate, the captain of my soul."

Birth and death are common experiences to all of us. We as physicians can help relieve pain sometimes and prolong life sometimes, but we cannot "make a person get well." It was some time before I understood this to the extent I understand it now. The patient must have a desire to get well—some reason or purpose. He must have a goal that animates and lifts him above the pain and duress. If this is not there, then we as physicians must make the effort to instill it. The reasons are whatever he makes them. Raising a family, writing a book, watching a grandchild grow, cultivating a garden, being the best of what he is—whether it's a cobbler of shoes or a leader of people.

In medical school we were told not to make friends with our patients but keep an objective distance. The longer I practice the more I see how wrong this is. For without an abiding interest and love there can be no true healing.

We must be physicians and friends. We must let the patient know we care through a hug or a reassuring touch. We as doctors have a holy trust. Holy is the root of the word holistic. By performance it has come to signify the whole person—body, mind and spirit. We have no true healing unless we deal with the whole. In holistic medicine, the spirit is the life, the mind the builder, and the physical the result. Our job is to access the physician within the patient. We want patients to get involved. We help them to make the most reasonable and enlightened choices.

Having deified doctors since childhood, some patients may at first fear taking responsibility. Simple meditation can open up the subconscious mind and supplement any other treatment that is indicated. In meditation, patients begin to realize that they have an identity apart from their disease. They get in touch with their divine spirit and are reminded of their connection to the universe. This is our universe. We didn't come into the world by accident, nor does our life stretch out by accident. We belong here.

Little miracles take place all the time. I'm not a great sports fan, but I was intrigued by the spontaneous recovery of a football star who had injured his leg so badly just before the 1995 play-offs, that team doctors and specialists had said that the football season would be long over before he could play again. The player's name was Reggie White and he was rated one of the best linemen in the history of the Green Bay Packers. The fans in Green Bay were distraught. What chance did they have in the approaching play-offs without this stalwart player? But they underestimated Reggie and his affiliation with the Lord.

Reggie got down on his prayer bones and asked the Lord to help, not for himself, but for the thousands of loyal fans and for his teammates who were crestfallen by this blow to the team. The pain had been agonizing, and it was an effort to sit down, get up or take a step. It looked hopeless. But Reggie had prayed before with good results and he wasn't discouraged. Reggie was also an ordained minister, and the Lord had been his physician within for some time.

Two or three days after he had been counted out, Reggie stood up without pain, and walked around his house, free and easy. He tested the injured leg—no pain. His doctors could only shake their heads. The injury was one that normally would have taken months to heal. The Green Bay coach had been disconsolate and he couldn't believe it when told about the transformation. Reggie called on him that same day, at midnight, to let the coach see for himself that Reggie was ready to play. "I owe it all to the Lord," he said. And he might have added, "to the physician within," who happened to be the Lord in this case.

The healing process is not all that mysterious. Every cell in the body has an innate intelligence which subconsciously links it with the healing process. When we cut or bruise a hand, a healing takes place without any conscious effort on our part. The blood coagulates, getting a message from the brain. A protective scab forms. As the wound heals, the scab drops off. The hand is as good as new. Through meditation and visualization we induce a similar healing process in various parts of the body that don't normally heal spontaneously.

We train patients with biofeedback to extend the subconscious mind's power to the physician within. To lose gobs of fat, for instance, the patient can visualize himself shedding weight in the desert sun. Or, to eliminate an asthmatic condition, imaging his lungs as floating wings of oxygen. At the same time, the patient may pursue a disciplined diet, exercise or take conventional medication. Patients frequently transpose me, an obvious image, into their subconscious meditations as their inner physician, reinforcing the treatment I have consciously given. This is another example of the potency of the subconscious mind, with the individual taking charge of his treatment and connecting with his body.

We often look back to look ahead. Jesus sent his disciples out on their own, giving each an independent mission. He was saying that there is a time in our lives when we need no longer be disciples. At that point we accept the responsibility for who and what we are. This is what we work with in patients. To make them part of the healing process. No longer are they disciples who do what they are told to do. That is when it becomes a challenge—when they must come to grips with the person they see in the mirror every day and consider what influenced their illness. In doing this many of us define our relationship with God, wondering about things that people have always wondered about.

At 14, I wondered about the universality of this great unknown. I remember asking my missionary father how a loving God could condemn people who had never heard of Him—like the natives we encountered in the jungles of India when we traveled village to village bringing medical care and the gospel. This question is as important to me now as it was then. My father answered, "Gladys, you have enough work to do in this life, making sure that you're doing what God wants you to do. That should keep you busy for your whole life. Let God take care of the other children he has created." It may have been a very wise answer. Without it, I would have kept asking questions for which there was no rational explanation—at least not one my father might have given me. Yet as I grew older and came to my parents' country, now my country, and went on to medical school, my faith in a bountiful God grew as I participated in the never-ending miracle of babies' births. How could a mere human being like myself produce a child with a molecular structure more complex than any machine the most brilliant scientist could devise? A baby is a gift of God. What else could this precious bundle of life be, with its everlasting promise of the continuity of life?

I see God's presence every day. In the miracles of life, in the wonders of nature, in this great land with its diversity of people and in the miracle of healing. I see God when I see a life that has almost been extinguished regain its spark as though God had touched the person with a magic wand and made him well. In trying to understand this divine intervention, we sometimes find it convenient to put God in boxes. I remember a sermon our Presbyterian minister gave when my children were young. The title was, "Is God a Presbyterian?"

It was a good question, as it got us thinking about what God was. In trying to make our relationship to God real, there is always the temptation to expand on that reality and to try to make it "fit" with our points of view. As a physician I have had no trouble with making God "fit." I have patients who are born-again Christians, who are strict Catholics, who are Moslems, who are Buddhists, who are Hindus, who are Jews and who are plain old down-the-road Presbyterians or Methodists. It seems to me that my job in working with them—as a physician and also as a counselor—is not to try and make them understand my philosophy or my relationship to God, but for me to try to understand theirs if I am going to be of any help.

This frequently means stretching myself beyond my own philosophical point of view and allowing my patients to be exactly who they are and respecting them for that. Respect and love and healing go hand in hand, and if I'm going to be an instrument for God's healing, then I need to allow myself to be used the way my patients need to have me used. One thing that I learned from my father was that I can't change anybody else. I might want to influence them. I might pray for them. I might love them. I might even bully them a little bit, but I can't change them. If I can be clear enough and loving enough and respect myself enough so that God will use me as an instrument of his healing, then I may be able to have an influence on another person's life and help them change. But never, never can I make them change. I can't say it too often: The patient's will is supreme. No physician should forget that.

I love to sit in my meditation garden when I have a few moments and watch the natural world unfold. There is so much to see and learn. One evening I observed a flock of wild geese fly over very high in the sky, very definitely in their V position with the lead goose setting a leisurely pace. Contrary to what I had always believed, the lead goose in this formation was not the strongest goose but the weakest, and with good reason. If the weakest goose were in the rear, it would soon be left behind. If the strongest goose were up front, it might set a pace which the others, particularly the weakest goose, couldn't maintain. The weaker lead goose set a slower pace that everyone could maintain. And the stronger geese in the rear were able, with their wings, to create air currents that would support the slower geese and help them along.

I was struck not only by the wisdom of these creatures but by the concern for the weaker members of their flock. It made a big impression on me and I have never forgotten it. As I thought about it further, I realized this pattern had parallels in our own lives, especially with the weak parts of our own bodies.

If, for instance, the weakest part of a body is the knee, then all the rest of the body has to pay attention to that knee and support it. It becomes the organ that sets the pace, the direction and the way the rest of the body goes. The lead organ can change, but it is still the one which gets the attention. As we focus on this most vulnerable of our organs, the rest of the body supports it and helps bring healing to it. As healing is brought to that organ, we find that the other parts of the body are also healed.

I am constantly amazed by the divine order that has put all of this together in such a rational way. It is an order that the great Albert Einstein, a reputed atheist, translated into a mathematical equation. Einstein's views on the deity were a matter of great debate at Princeton where he was a scientist in residence. But only the young would have dared step where others feared to tread. The son of a Princeton professor, who had been granted a 16th-birthday wish, requested a meeting with Einstein. With the candor of youth he asked the world-renowned scientist, "Why is it, sir, that you don't believe in God?"

Einstein replied without lifting an eyebrow, "I'm not so sure we have a difference, young man. I see a supreme order in the world. You call this order God."

The Miracle
of Birth

*Before I formed thee in
the belly, I knew thee.*

—JEREMIAH 1:5

L ife is a continuous, never-ending miracle
which begins with the greatest miracle of
all—the baby. I see the wisdom of the ages in a
child's innocent stare as it makes an instant connection with the family circle into which it is
introduced. I have seen babies at three months
who wouldn't let anyone touch or hold them
but the father and mother. I have seen others
who reach out to apparent strangers and greet
them with the affection of a remembered past.
We know of babies who, before they could
speak, have vivid dreams of people and places.
Later, when they can talk, they verbally recall, to

the amazement of their parents, the details of these dreams. They are called precocious or imaginative. But none of these labels explain why these images may have brimmed to the surface.

At the Scottsdale Holistic Medical Group, our wellness program begins with the first stirring of life inside the mother's body. We acquaint the mother with the child she is bearing, a child different from any other in the universe. We help the two get to know each other and to understand that they are bound in body, mind and spirit. I have observed this unique union on countless occasions, sensing that whatever subconscious communication there is before birth may very well transcend conscious connection after birth.

We now know that whatever affects the mother has a corollary impact on the embryonic child, whether it be an unhappy marriage or the stress of being unmarried and unloved. The child knows, above all, whether it is wanted or unwanted, and if the latter feeling is strong enough, the child may find a way to leave its unhappy home and return at a more favorable time.

We also know, only too well, that an addictive parent can pass on her addiction to the sensitive fetus, along with physical and mental defects. So it is not surprising that whatever the mother thinks or feels should also impact an embryonic body and mind.

There appears to be a new breed of child. They speak like old souls at the age of two or three, seeming totally familiar with their surroundings and insisting that they have come into a world not all that new to them.

I have colleagues, like Dr. Jean Chapman, a former medical director of Ford Motors and Rockwell International, who share my interest in children who appear to know better than adults do how and why they got here. Chapman, like myself, has delivered hundreds of babies, guiding them through their infancy as they claimed their place in the family. Chapman is intrigued by the fact that so many "New Age" babies appear to arrive at just the right time, adding a special dimension to a family that almost seems predestined.

She goes on to explain further. "It was as though they knew everyone before they arrived in the home, making the kind of spontaneous comments as soon as they could talk that made you wonder if they had been in any of these homes before.

"The comments were often significant and direct, sometimes sentimental, as they popped out of these childish mouths. Their language was plain. They spoke in accents of authority, with a detail they could not have consciously conceived. They spoke with reproach at having been turned away, with reminders of a stunning nature to mothers with a hidden past.

"What they had to say was usually blurted out without any childish design for attention, like 'That's not the way it was last time,' from a two-year-old who made the announcement with a solemn face. Or sometimes they'll say in a half-accusing voice while being chided by the mother, 'You said you wouldn't do that anymore.'"

Chapman began to ask herself questions like, "Is reincarnation truly a possibility? If so, do we choose our parents?" It reminded her of the story of the biblical Elizabeth who recognized the God-given baby in her cousin Mary's womb, when the baby she herself was bearing moved inside her. And had not the Lord told the prophet Jeremiah, "Before I formed thee in the belly I knew thee." Apparently, the Jeremiah of the Bible had existed before and was known to God, if to no other.

The scientifically schooled Chapman was a born skeptic, however. Bible stories notwithstanding, she needed more than a few random words from a few random children to make a believer of her. Then, from out of nowhere, a very intriguing event occurred in her own family. This happened some years ago, as Chapman explains it.

"My son was then three and a half. We were talking about what fantastic times we had playing together. We had just been in a skiing area and were driving home. I said offhandedly, giving him a little pat, 'I sure wish you had come into my life sooner. Think of all the fun we've missed.'

"He lifted his bright little face and his eyes were like saucers. Very solemnly, with a wistful look, he announced, 'Well, I tried twice before but you weren't ready, so I had to go back.'"

The mother's hands gripped the wheel. It was as though a thunderbolt had struck. A number of thoughts raced through her mind. She remembered the children she had listened to when she was working with babies. Then a second mystifying thought flashed through her mind. How had this child of hers known something that no one but she knew?

"What," she said, "are you saying?"

He looked at her patiently as if trying to make her understand what he knew only too well. "Well, you weren't ready," he said in that grownup way of his, "so I had to wait."

She marveled as her mind went back in time: "No friends, no relatives, not even my spouse—no one—was aware that I'd had two miscarriages."

She was in for another start while traveling in India with me some fifteen years later. An astrologer at the Taj Mahal insisted on reading her life history from her birth chart. At first he frowned. "You do not have children," he said. Then he amended his statement. "No, no, you have one. And you almost had two others."

She left it at that. Her son had said all that had to be said.

Chapman's experience was no surprise to me. I had dealt with a generation of children in the '80s and '90s who talked about the mommies they had revisited as if they were talking about Santa Claus or Alice in Wonderland in a world not all that strange to them. In one instance, this normally withdrawn child had attached herself to a younger woman, an apparent stranger, who had casually called on the child's parents. The visitor was strangely moved when the six-year-old girl climbed on her lap and announced she wanted to leave with her.

"I know her," little Jamie said. "We belong together." She turned to her mother. "Is it all right?"

It wasn't all right.

The parents apologized, and with a laugh said, "Jamie says the oddest things at times."

Jamie followed the visitor to the door, tears filling her eyes as the woman stopped for a moment to hug and kiss her. She, too, had tears in her eyes. "Please come back," the child said. "You promised."

The incident may have been a childish quirk. Yet it left a lasting impression and sent the mind of the visitor whirling back in years to the time she had self-induced an abortion. She still carried the painful memory. Would she have had a little daughter like this? She might never know. They would have been the same age. She sighed, and the tears again came to her eyes. She was compulsively drawn to Jamie, but it could have been any child that age, she told herself. Could it be some sort of retribution? It seemed unlikely. She thought she had hurt no one but herself, but now she wondered if that was true. And she would go on wondering.

I have heard similar stories many times, and it was an issue I had struggled with for many years. I had six children of my own, and I was one of five. I would never have thought of an abortion for myself. I saw people I liked and respected, including doctors, on both sides of the question, and they were people who had not lightly come to such diverse views.

Once a longtime patient came in with an unusual and enigmatic story. She had been having lunch with her four-year-old daughter when little Dottie said out of nowhere, "Do you know,

Mommy, you weren't always my mommy?" The mother, Phyllis, smiled and patted the child's head, thinking this some childish sport that the little girl was having with her. She saw soon enough that the child was serious. Her blue eyes were opened wide, and she had a grave look on her pretty face.

The mother decided to play it out like a game. "So when wasn't I your mommy, my dear?"

"The last time." Her little face screwed up in a frown. "But it wasn't really the last time, Mommy. There was another time."

The mother sat back in her chair, not knowing how to respond.

"I had a different mommy then," the child went on. She mentioned the woman's name. It was nobody Phyllis knew, nor was it a name she was familiar with.

Phyllis figured it was all a child's fantasy and she thought she'd humor her daughter. They had finished with lunch by this time. "So what was the last time, dear?"

The child pursed her lips. "The last time, Mommy, was when I was four inches long and I was in your tummy. But Daddy wasn't ready to be my daddy yet. He wasn't ready to marry you. And so I went away."

A tremor went through the mother. There had been an abortion at a time when the fetus would have been that size. But no one had known about it except the father. She married him two years later when his divorce from another woman was eventually finalized.

As all this spilled out of Phyllis, we looked at each other, different thoughts running through our minds. The mother thought of her love for the daughter who she felt had returned as a blessing of the Lord, almost like a tale out of old Scripture. I sat quietly for a few moments, pondering the implications of what I had just been told. I knew my patient well enough to realize she had not fabricated the story. So what did it mean?

Obviously, the child had something to say about what had gone on. Here she was telling her mother about an abortion she should have known nothing about—and the reasons for it, which were true. In the child's mind, there was no problem, because she was able to come back and she seemed content to be where she was. As for the mother, she gladly accepted Dottie as the daughter she had lost.

Some years later, when the daughter was almost 17, the mother, still youngish at 40, had a tubal ligation to prevent pregnancy. She was menstruating at an age when she thought bearing children would be a disservice to a child and a strain on the family.

There was an ironic development which the mother disclosed during a subsequent physical examination. She and her daughter usually menstruated on the first of the month. This month, Phyllis menstruated as usual, but Dottie, now 17, missed her period. She was pregnant and not married, and the young man had gone off.

Phyllis's mind flew back over the years to the conversation with four-year-old Dottie. "My husband and I talked about our daughter's pregnancy and felt in our heart of hearts that we could accept the child with love if Dottie wished to bring the child into our family. We wanted to give her an alternative. The thought of a child after what she had been through warmed our hearts. But the decision had to be Dottie's."

To their disappointment, Dottie, with no love for an absent father, opted for an abortion. That week Phyllis missed her period and had a dream that turned out to be prophetic.

"In this dream I was on the top floor of a three-story house. I followed a young man down the outside stairs to the bottom which was on the ocean. I saw an infant being carried out to sea on the top of a wave. I ran after it into the surf and scooped it up in my arms and brought it up on the sand. The dream was in color. Blue."

A week later Phyllis had a pregnancy test, not thinking for a moment that it would be positive. To the surprise of both this woman with a tubal ligation and her middle-aged husband, the test revealed she was pregnant. She was in a state of shock. "It was like an altered state of consciousness. My mind constantly reverted to the luncheon with Dottie when she was four, and to the law of retribution."

Having a psychic nature, with the ability to foresee things for others from time to time, Phyllis went into her subconscious mind in an attempt to put everything in place. She realized that life did have its day of reckoning.

"I saw where I had had my abortion and then Dottie had come back to me. Though she was a child, she was understanding and gladly accepted her place in the family. Now, with her child aborted, I understood—as Dottie had long before—the desire for the unborn child to find a place in the family. This time, he came back to a grandmother who was happy to take him in. I say 'him' because the color blue in my dream had foreshadowed a boy."

The thwarted grandmother was now an expectant mother. She gave birth to a boy, and she had no doubt that it was the daughter's fetus, maneuvering his spirit in such a way that he would stay in the family.

Had the child decided for himself? How else could it have happened? Had a Higher Power somehow intervened? It gave me a new perspective on the unseen hand that sometimes governs our most intimate actions.

I sometimes think God is also watching over pregnant teenagers who are babies themselves. So often they are 13, 14, 15, yes and even 11 or 12 years old. At the clinic we had a 15-year-old girl, pretty and precocious. She came from what is commonly known as a good family and something of this nature was wholly unexpected. Marriage was out of the question and the family was confused about what should be done. I suggested that they pray and make a decision. Father, mother and the rest of the family all came to the same, reluctant decision: abortion.

I had negative feelings about abortion, even when they seemed necessary, and I had been hoping for a spontaneous miscarriage. What with all the prayers for the best possible solution, I had added my own prayers.

On the eve of the arranged abortion I got a call from the family. There was a relieved note in the voice of the girl's mother. The girl had aborted spontaneously, without any difficulty or effort.

In other situations like this, I've often asked the young women to write down their reasons for the abortion and their feelings against abortion. I ask them to make the best decision for all concerned in as unemotional a way as they can. I am surprised how many of these girls stick it out and decide to have the baby.

We know that the child and mother are in subtle communication before birth. They are one and the same flesh, on the same wavelength, and it is never too soon to establish a spiritual bond between them. I tell the mother to communicate with this entity waiting to be born, to let the baby know it is loved and wanted. And if this is one of those circumstances where there is an obstacle, the mother needs to let the unborn child know what it is.

I still have a problem with women who want an abortion for convenience, to avoid embarrassment or a threat to the stability of a marriage. Children have a right to be born if they want to be, or to abort themselves rather than come into a home where they aren't wanted. While this may seem a novel idea, it happens. I remember with dismay a 12-year-old pregnant by her father. There was no way I could counsel that child to give birth. To my relief and to the family's, the girl aborted spontaneously.

A spontaneous miscarriage reflects an agreement between the unborn but sentient fetus and the mother. It sometimes removes the guilt of abortion. It's important that the unborn baby not feel that the unready mother doesn't love it, and that the child understand that it may find a better home one day when the time is right.

As a child of India, I was aware of the Eastern belief in reincarnation, and despite my early Christian experience, and the Christ-consciousness guiding me then and now, I thought often about it. I had read what Voltaire had once said: "It is just as remarkable to have been born once as twice." The birth of a child was indeed a miracle of creation, and creation, as the province of the Lord, had no limitations. So why not a born-again child?

As the concept of the continuity of life grew into reality in my mind, the pieces began to fall in place. Was it possible that we have no beginning or end as spiritual creatures? Can we choose our parents? Are these experiences that develop our growth and understanding? And, as Jesus said, is death but the prelude to everlasting life?

Birthing babies was my special delight. I exulted in the renewal of life. Each birth was an adventure and each was so different. But they were all a never-ending miracle. I had no doubt that the child had a mind of its own. Yet in all the struggle between the pro-choice and pro-life factions, no one seemed interested in what the child thought.

Of course there are times when a woman feels she can't handle a pregnancy—because of rape, incest, poverty, illness or a disinterested father. Nevertheless, many of these mothers never consider abortion. One young mother I knew was horrified by the thought. She had nothing to fall back on—no money, no family, no man to turn to. She kept sending messages to the baby inside her, telling him she loved him, but it would be better for him if he moved on now, and came back at another, more auspicious time.

She was confused. Was she, who had been abandoned herself, abandoning her child? She left it up to him.

After this decision a deep calm settled over her.

"That evening in bed," she confided, "I was able to move my consciousness down to my uterus. It felt like a cavernous, secure shelter. In a rather suspended yet elevated space, this soul and I had some serious communication. It felt completely natural. I explained that it wasn't the right time for me to become a mother. With love I let him know that it had nothing to do with him. I urged him to find another mother. The following day I passed a blood clot and soon resumed my regular periods. I had perceived him as a boy and gave him the name 'Richard.'"

She made an appointment with a doctor, a medical doctor who believed the soul was immortal. "He confirmed my miscarriage, then did a spiritual clearing to send Richard on. I released him with love."

She eventually married, telling herself she had only postponed the birth and Richard would return as the same soul one day. Years later, she met a young man who she was sure was her son. He was the right age and had the same name. There was instant communication. The first day they met he called her "Mom," and she felt a mother's love. It was so easy and natural. When she said his name, he smiled and pressed her hand as though he remembered. They saw each other whenever they could. There was always the same warm feeling. But it never quite fell into place. How could it? It was out of place—and time. Too much had happened in between and they were no longer the same people.

There is always something different in these stories of spontaneous miscarriages, something new to learn and to marvel about in the angry division over what is best for "baby."

There are times when a child may remember what a mother has forgotten. This mother I knew had three pregnancies and two daughters. A year after her older girl, Ann, was born, Alice, the mother, became pregnant again. In the second month of her pregnancy, she slipped and fell on a stone ramp. It was a hard fall, but the pain passed and she felt fine. But from that point on the fetus didn't develop. Her doctor questioned his diagnosis, saying she may not have been pregnant, but at five months she proved him wrong: She aborted spontaneously.

Four months later Alice became pregnant with her second daughter. Everything went well. She delivered a healthy nine-pound girl. She had been hoping for a boy to round out the family, but she greeted the birth rapturously and fondled the baby girl, Mary, as though she knew her. "I found myself saying things like, 'I didn't know they would let you be my baby.'" "They" were the good Lord and the angels.

She often felt that little Mary was like a younger sister, a playmate with adult understandings. "At times, this younger daughter seemed like an old soul, someone who had gone on, then returned to our little family."

As time passed, Alice continued to be intrigued by this chumminess. She enjoyed talking with the girls about their early childhood. She mentioned the desire she originally had for a boy the second time, but also said how delighted she was that her little Mary had arrived after her miscarriage.

One day, the family was driving home from a little trip. Mary had been sitting in the back seat, so quiet that the mother thought she had fallen asleep. Suddenly she blurted out, "No, Mama, it wasn't a miscarriage. I killed it."

The mother turned, startled, "Killed what, dear?"

"Your baby, Mama. The one you lost."

The mother smiled at this childish fantasy.

"No, honey, I fell. Don't you remember my telling you about it once? It was an accident."

The child shook her head. "No, Mama. It was a boy, what you wanted. I wanted to be a girl and to be your little sister."

Alice drove on quietly, in virtual shock. The girl had spoken so casually that it seemed the implications had been lost on her.

"I tried to reassure her," Alice later told me, "telling her she had nothing to do with it, that miscarriages occurred fairly frequently after a bad fall. She didn't seem at all concerned. She was very much alive, still my child." She smiled. "And all girl."

With my background, plus having a minister son and daughter-in-law, I am sympathetic to young mothers with strong religious convictions who are troubled by the prospect of another child. One impassioned mother I knew had two babies in two years. She felt stretched out, but abortion was never an option. She had run the gamut of belief systems, hellfire-and-damnation Southern Baptist to tightly-bound Catholic to a God-centered awareness. None had given her the support she was looking for.

She had married for love at 19, and had her first child at 20. She was a strict Catholic, having converted from the Baptist Church. She had a second child at 21. She was barely out of her teens, married to a lapsed Catholic trying to build a career, and she was appalled at the possibility of a dozen children by the time she was 30. "I pathetically tried to practice the rhythm system advocated by my church," she said, "but it didn't seem to work for me."

Her faith was strong, but her awareness was limited by her inability to practice the rhythm method correctly. "The first time my husband and I had relations after the second baby's birth, I became pregnant—after three months of waiting to have a period again and then three months of taking my temperature before we could express ourselves sexually. I was 22, he was 23. In three years of marriage, with two full-term pregnancies, we had abstained more than we had enjoyed a sexual relationship. To add to my distress, I knew I would be violently ill from the end of the fourth week to the end of the 12th week, as I had been before.

"I felt betrayed by my faith, by the church and by God. I felt righteously indignant. I went into a church and knelt at the communion rail. I can't remember if others were present. What I do remember is the depth of my emotions running through every cell of my body. I felt a blind rage seething inside me. I beat on the padded rail, crying, 'I kept my part of the bargain. You didn't keep yours.' I pointed a finger at the tabernacle. 'I won't have an abortion because it is a mortal sin. But I expect you to take care of it. I cannot carry another baby so soon. We can't afford another one now.' I literally ordered the God of the tabernacle to abort the baby."

Too angry to be appalled by the challenge she had flung out, she managed to compose herself and said calmly, "I'll cheerfully accept the child given to me after a rest—at least a year without a pregnancy." And then she strode out of the church, half-wondering whether she'd be punished for this affront to God and the church.

She could do nothing now but wait and pray. "I did not experience nausea with that third pregnancy. That in itself seemed like a miracle and a thrill ran through me. Maybe somebody was listening. Maybe God was smiling at me, wherever he was, looking down on us poor mortals who have so much trouble knowing what he wants of us.

"Only a few weeks later, two and a half months into the pregnancy, I spontaneously aborted. In spite of all my raving, or because of it, I had been heard. I had not cried out in vain."

She had some qualms. "I asked the doctor whether it had been a boy or girl. He couldn't tell as the fetus had stopped developing close to the fourth week, which was the time I had gone into the church and asked the Almighty for help. There was no doubt in my mind that God had answered my prayers. I had asked God—and the church—for a year's rest. And I was prepared to meet my share of the bargain.

"Little more than a year later I became pregnant again. I guess God really listened to me that day, and kept me honest. I knew somehow the child was going to be a girl, and I'd jokingly remind her, patting my tummy occasionally, that she was the answer to the bargain I had made.

"Two years after my miscarriage I gave birth to my third daughter, a healthy, smiling, wonderful gift of God. I called her Grace."

As the child grew up, they discussed whether Grace was the soul who made the hasty exit and later came back. "She decided not, as she is a fiery Sagittarius who could not imagine herself as an ambiguous Gemini or a misty Cancer. I didn't much care. I felt I had my daughter back."

The communication between a mother and the child inside her has never ceased to intrigue me. The experiences I heard about were varied and heartwarming, revealing a depth of understanding and love that transcends the usual family affections—and often brought out a resourcefulness that many young people never realized they had. A war and the separation from the young man she loved tested the strength and resolve of one young woman I knew who had just finished high school and was ready for college.

Not until Susan's young man had gone off to war did this teenager realize she was pregnant. She didn't panic.

"I thought of writing and letting him know, but there was nothing he could do. He had enough to handle in the middle of a war so far from home. I knew I'd have to handle it alone somehow. I couldn't tell my parents. They would have been distressed, and what could they do? I was 17, planning to enter college in a few weeks. I could hardly turn up on campus in a maternity dress. And I wouldn't get an abortion. The very thought was repugnant to me."

As her family physician, I was aware of Susan's background. She had manifested some psychic sensitivity as a child, remembering in detail the circumstances of her birth and delivery, and frequently being able to predict little things in the lives of friends. She was also a communicator, and she felt that the child beginning to live in her body would be a little girl—she never thought of it as a fetus. One day she decided she would talk to her and take the child into her confidence. She spoke softly, with tenderness, placing her hands on her stomach. She explained the situation, about Daddy having to go away, and about herself having to go to school. It was the wrong time to have a child. "I want you to know I love you, and that you will only be away a little while. We will be together again. I promise."

She believes the baby inside her must have listened. Into her third month, without any overt action on her part, she had a miscarriage. It was clean and without incident. She felt sad and wept, but told herself the child would be back—the same little girl she had lost.

She had not mentioned her pregnancy to anyone, not even to her best friend, Fran, who was married and was two or three years older. Two years later to the day after Susan's miscarriage, Fran gave birth to a little girl. That same night, Susan was awakened from a fitful sleep by a child's voice saying, "Mama, I'm coming back."

"I had been tossing all night. Usually I slept very well. As I heard the child's voice I jumped out of bed. I could almost feel her presence. I had half-expected something like this. I had been wishing and hoping. But when it happened I still wasn't prepared, and I marveled at the wonder of it all. A thrill of joy swept over me. In that moment I knew it was my little girl—a promise fulfilled.

"I could hardly wait to see her. Nobody thought anything of my rushing over to the hospital. I was 'family.'"

Susan took her first look at the baby, and she knew. "They say all babies look alike, but not this one. I was glad she had come back to Fran. Fran was happily married and they would be a family. I could look in and be part of that. Fran and I were that close."

The baby had opened her eyes and smiled. The smile wrung Susan's heart, but she just smiled back. Her baby had returned and was in good hands. This was all that mattered. It never occurred to Susan that she might be playing out a fantasy, not with the child's response.

The child was named Terry, a name Susan liked. She visited Fran and the baby every chance she had.

"From the beginning we had this special bond, like we both knew of our previous connection. I thought of her as my child. She would throw up her arms to greet me with the happiest smile. When she was able to toddle she would rush into my arms. I could see that Fran and her husband were amused."

The couple made little of it. Susan was family and Terry couldn't have made a better or more significant choice. It was their secret, one that Susan wouldn't divulge—not then.

When Terry was three, her mother was again pregnant and Susan was visiting. Terry, as usual, plopped herself in Susan's lap, and threw her arms around her, blowing her a kiss. Then, to the amazement of her parents, she ruffled her little brow and said to the young woman holding her:

"Do you remember when I was in your tummy?"

A silence fell over the room. Susan was the first to respond.

"No, honey," she said, "you were in your mother's tummy."

The child shook her head. "Not that first time."

A shiver ran down Susan's spine. She wanted to kiss and embrace the little girl in her arms, but she was conscious of the others. She could see the child was looking at her, waiting. And so she said, for want of anything better:

"What did you do in my tummy?"

A sad look came into the little girl's eyes. "I cried."

Susan felt a pang. "Why did you cry?"

"Because they said I couldn't stay. They said it wasn't the time. They pulled me back."

Fran and her husband looked on with amazement. They didn't know what to make of it. Susan's mind flashed back in time, her joy tinged with sorrow. She could see the child looking at her, wanting her to go on.

"Who were *they*?" Susan finally asked, not knowing what to expect.

"The same ones that brought me to you."

Susan held back a sigh. "How did they pull you back?"

"With a long silver cord." She dropped one tiny hand to her navel.

How could there be any doubt? There was none in Susan's mind or the child's. Susan looked around the room and could see that Fran and her husband were upset. "Not so much by my closeness with the little girl, but at the thought of reincarnation. It violated the tenets of their church and their own convictions."

There was never any trouble with the parents. Having known nothing of Susan's pregnancy, they had no idea what was going on in her heart. She loved Fran as a sister, and she had no problem with Terry being where she was and with whom she was. It seemed almost natural in the circumstances. She saw the child routinely and was always greeted with the same affection. Occasionally a quizzical look passed across the child's face, as if she wanted her to know she was keeping their secret. Susan saw things in the child that were in her. Terry was extraordinarily sensitive and appeared to have an almost psychic divination of people's thoughts and circumstances. When the mother, Fran, was expecting another child, Terry mentioned one day that it would be a boy. She said it flat out, no question about it.

Fran gave birth to her second child after a difficult pregnancy. It was a boy. He was born with a respiratory problem and not expected to live. It was touch and go. Susan looked after Terry during this critical period. When she told Terry she had a new baby brother, the child became agitated and shook her head. "Not yet," she said, "he isn't here yet."

Susan remembered that day very well. "In a way she was right. For the boy, hovering close to death, was lying unconscious in a hospital respirator. The doctors had given up on him. Fran had come home and was already mourning her loss when little Terry came bouncing into the room to announce that the baby was ready to come home. It was time to pick him up.

"This," Susan recalled, "upset Fran because the doctors had already told her there was no chance and they were about to turn off the respirator."

Terry kept smiling, repeating what she had just said. Fran left for the hospital, not sure what she would find. She entered the nursery with some trepidation. There in a crib she found her baby boy, wide-eyed and healthy. Two hours earlier, the nurses told her, just as Terry made her announcement, the baby had opened his eyes, infused with new life. It was a miracle.

The mother-love feelings between Susan and Terry never changed. When Terry was 18, Susan told her of the aborted pregnancy and the voice she heard the night of Terry's birth.

"She understood. She had always felt our strong bond and her mother-love for me. All she did was hug me with tears in her eyes. She didn't have to say anything. I didn't have to explain. It was something we had shared all these years. She didn't ask about the father. It was as though she knew that, like so many others, he had never come back."

It is an ongoing relationship. "I always know when Terry needs me and is in trouble. Though it was difficult to let her go, I did learn something, something that has helped me greatly: The soul survives and learns what it has to learn of a past that lives on."

As a mother of six I have always sensed the closeness and the spiritual tie between a mother and the baby inside her, waiting to be born. I find myself moved now by the thoughts of another young pregnant mother, Bobbie McGarey, the minister wife of my minister son, John, who had written this letter while in labor with her first child:

Whether this sweet baby makes its arrival today or whenever, I have learned a valuable lesson. This baby—although seemingly mine and part of me—is not mine, but rather a child of God. This is a time of introspection for me like no other. For I am not merely me, but part of the God-force at work. This baby who has grown within me and shared my body, my food, my oxygen, my breath—this baby even now is independent. I have no control over it. I cannot choose when precisely I want it to be born—a lesson for our lives together. I cannot choose its life path. I can guide and suggest and direct, but I can't protect from sorrow or know what will happen in life. I must now—before it is born— accept it as a child of God and give the control to God. My faith is stretched in this situation like never before. I hang on a cord of trust which is God. As my baby lives on a cord within me.

And so she ends:

We'll find some laughter waiting
We'll find some sorrow, too
But as our journey keeps on moving
All our dreams we'll give to you.

Gifts from God

*O*ut of the mouths of babes . . .

—THE BOOK OF PSALMS 8:2

After listening to so many stories of mothers who induced spontaneous abortions it was refreshing to know there were children who wanted to come into this murky world of ours and mothers who wanted them.

I knew many of these mothers. As a doctor whose special delight had always been babies, I had some insight into births that were not only a blessing but something of a miracle. One reminding me of the birth of the Old Testament prophet Samuel to an older Hannah, because of her prayers and her dedication of the infant to the service of the Lord. This mother, Veronica, unlike Hannah, never had a vision in her life, and had been praying for a child for years.

Veronica felt abandoned by the Lord. She didn't know why she couldn't become pregnant. She loved her husband. They had a good marriage. She was healthy enough, young enough, willing enough. She had all kinds of tests which proved inconclusive. Low in spirits, Veronica wondered why there were so many women having children they didn't want, when her heart's desire was denied her.

On the night before Thanksgiving, Veronica left the hospital after having undergone more tests. She felt empty inside—bereft and childless still. To make matters worse, her husband was several hours late picking her up. When he finally arrived, he had to immediately drop her off at a bowling alley-restaurant while he went back to work.

Veronica told me, "I felt so alone. As though the Lord had forsaken me, denying me my birthright as a woman. I was not a crybaby, but I found myself choking back my tears. I had three hours to wait in this dreary restaurant, which was separated from the bowling lanes by an open wrought-iron barrier. I was sipping a cup of coffee when I became aware of a child standing on the other side of the barrier. He looked to be about two years old, but rather small for his age, and had a Buster Brown haircut. A light shone on him from the ceiling. He looked at me pensively through the wrought-iron bars, almost as though he knew me. Finally he spoke. "'You're in jail.'"

"I smiled. With the bars it did look something like a jail. I was surprised but I went along with him.

"'No, I'm not,'" I said, "'you are.'"

"He looked around, taking in just about everything. 'The whole world's in a jail.'

"That seemed a strange thing for a little child to say. I was more and more intrigued. 'Who's going to let us out?' I asked.

"He was very matter-of-fact. 'God will.'

"What did this tiny tot know of God? I was beginning to wonder if it was all a dream, forgetting, meanwhile, how depressed I'd been.

"'And who's going to ask him for the key?'" I said, carrying it along.

"At this, he cocked his head, as though thinking about it. Then with a radiant smile said, 'I'll ask God to let you out.'"

Suddenly, Veronica took heart. She felt there was a message there for her brought by the small child "I felt like the weight of the world had been lifted from my shoulders," she told me. "I was free to be whatever I wanted. I looked up to say something and realized he was gone. I pinched myself. It was all so real. I looked for him but didn't find him. No one else had seen him. He seemed to have disappeared into thin air. Had I imagined it all? I didn't see how, since I remembered the conversation as plain as day. It occurred to me it could have been a vision, like the visions in the Bible when people ask God for help. Quite often an angel would appear. Could this little boy be an angel? I didn't say anything about it to my husband when he came by to pick me up. He would have thought I was crazy, overwrought by my desire for a child."

The next few weeks Veronica walked on air. Her depression had left her. She didn't bother with any more tests. She kept seeing the boy, as though she could reach out and touch him. She loved the way he looked at her, and marveled at how well he had spoken. She may have imagined it, but it was as real as anything she had ever known. She had a feeling God had heard her prayers and her spirits soared.

Two months later she conceived. Like Hannah, who had prayed to the Lord, her womb had opened and she was to have a child.

In the ninth month Veronica gave birth to a beautiful baby boy. It was an easy birth and the child was delivered without complications. He gave her a smile, and nodded off to sleep.

She thought of the bowling alley-restaurant encounter often. Then some three years after her experience—three years and three months precisely—she dropped into the place with her son for lunch. He was 28 months old.

She told me, "It was very nice. We ate and Bobby played on the floor with a toy car he had brought along. He dropped it through the bars and I went around to get it. As I stood up I looked at him. He was watching me through the bars. I had a strong feeling of déjà vu, as if I had been through all this before. He looked at me with eyes that had the glint of a smile, and said in a quiet voice, 'Bless you, Mom.'

"In that instant, I realized that he was the child I saw some three years before. He was small for his age and spoke very well. And his haircut was the same. I remembered now how casually he spoke of God, asking God for a key to let me out, to free me, to take me out of the prison I had made for myself. Suddenly I reached out and gave him a big hug. I couldn't help myself. He smiled, just like he had that day. I realized in that instant the day of miracles was not over. There was still a God who listened and he had sent my little boy to me."

And so he had, for children are gifts from God, though only a few remember.

I recall what a friend, Rabbi Herbert Weiner, a student of the Kabbala, said. "In the ancient wisdom of the Jewish faith there was a belief that before one was born he was given the opportunity to view everything that was going to happen to him in his next lifetime. Then the Angel of Forgetfulness touches him gently on the upper lip. And he forgets everything he saw, and he is born."

This generation of babies is a constant delight. They have such lively imaginations and seem devoid of fear. So often, as we've seen, they remember vividly events before they were born. Others remember dreams they had when only a few weeks old. Where had the dreams come from?

After surgery this one girl kept insisting she had to go back to the recovery room. The nurse reassured her there was no need to go back. "You're doing fine."

"I must," said the girl.

"Why?" said the nurse.

"To tell all those people they're not going to die."

She disappeared. The nurse checked it out. Several semi-conscious patients told of a young girl who floated by and stopped at their beds, touching them, telling them they were going to get well. And they got well. All described her alike—a slip of a girl with dark eyes that seemed to go through them, and a face like an angel. It was the same girl.

Nothing God does surprises me. He created the whole universe. Why should he have trouble creating little children with increased sensitivity for the critical days ahead?

We have to deal with life as we find it. There's no better place to start but the beginning. Because of a baby's sensitivity, what the parents think, say and do during pregnancy not only impacts who that child is, but how it lives out its life. The music we listen to, the TV shows we watch, the emotions we work with during the pregnancy, all these have an affect on the soul just as the food we eat, the exercise we do, and the material things we deal with. If we spend a good deal of time in prayer, the soul coming in knows that. If we listen to good music the soul responds to that. Research with ultrasound techniques has shown that most babies will draw away from hardrock music. Soft or classical music is something they enjoy and respond to positively.

Medically, we are acutely aware of physical things. Smoking, drugs, alcohol, all impact the well-being of the unborn baby. Emotions and spiritual attitudes have their impact. We have many examples of the pregnant mother's thinking on the baby's health. The mother can make the difference.

One mother, Sandy, was having a difficult time. She thought she might lose her child. She had a placenta previa, which meant that the placenta was moving across the opening of the uterus, already partially blocking it. She was already bleeding and would most likely go into premature labor. Sandy was going to have to stay in bed to reduce the bleeding, hopefully carry the baby another month or so and then have a C-section (Caesarean).

She had been told by one doctor that nothing else could be done. We gave her an alternative. I suggested she use a castor oil pack over her abdomen and visualize the placenta moving away from the cervix up along the uterine wall. She had an active physician within working for her as well as a physician outside. She understood this very well, and was able to bring her mind into play. She became mentally involved, excited by the thought of helping herself.

She talked to the baby and to the placenta, controlled by her mind and that of the child's, the two being joined. She visualized the placenta moving up and away from the cervix into the uterine cavity. Three weeks later the ultrasound revealed that the placenta had moved from the mouth of the uterus. There was no longer any danger of a placenta previa. Sandy breathed a sigh of relief. Her spirits lifted. She proceeded to go to term and had a nine-pound baby boy.

Emotions are easily transmitted. So many children are affected by a mother's stress during pregnancy. Some years ago I had a patient, Mary, whose pregnancy seemed to be going along very well until she and her husband developed severe financial problems. As a result he became extremely depressed and ended up in a psychiatric unit. Mary appeared to be dealing very well with the trouble she was going through. As it turned out, however, she was keeping it all inside. Her concerns and emotions were so deep they were passed on to her baby. When the baby was born she looked extremely pale. Blood work disclosed that the baby was anemic. Despite all our efforts to heal her, three days after her birth the baby died. An autopsy showed that this newborn had seven stomach ulcers—the mother's emotions had so deeply impacted upon the baby. The subconscious mind had the power to heal—or kill. The baby testified to that—with her life.

Since so much of a child's well-being depends on its entrance into life, I stress the method of birth should hinge wholly on the mother's needs. It is time for the pregnant woman to state how she wants her baby brought into the world. I like "my babies" born into the light, not darkness. When we die we are seeking the light. When we come into this world we have gone through a period of darkness and development in the womb. We are looking for the light on the outside. When I deliver a baby I see the child searching for the light. When their eyes move around and find the light they latch on to it. These are happy, smiling babies. Recently, after I delivered a baby I placed her in her mother's arms. The little girl looked into her mother's eyes and smiled. She was delivered naturally, without medication. The mother's first two children, delivered in the conventional medical way, had screamed as if in pain the first few hours after birth. We have become so engrossed in scientific technique we often forget that mother and baby are what it's all about.

Most mothers can deal with pain. The greatest problem is fear. The best support for a woman in labor is to ease her fears. Those around her should let her know that she has not been abandoned.

I have an idea babies have something to do with the time and place of their birth. I saw this with a boy born to a young couple who had moved to Arizona from the great Northwest.

There was no difficulty until the last six weeks of pregnancy. Sara, the mother, came into the office and I saw the baby was in breech position—opposite the normal vertex position with the head presenting first. I was able to rotate the breech so the head was down where it belonged. I told Sara to come back in a week, which she did every week thereafter. Each time, the baby was in breech and each time I turned it around.

When Sara went into labor she called me from home. I asked her to check the baby's position. She felt a lump under her ribs, which was the baby's head. I told her to talk to the baby in a loving way and see if she could get him to turn around again. She did this very easily, having watched me do it several times. They had good communication. By the time we met at the hospital the baby was fine and the delivery went well. The child delivered in the normal vertex position, the head presenting first.

The topsy-turvy days were over. Or so we thought.

Sara brought the baby in after a month for a checkup. She was upset because the baby seemed terrified of everything. He bawled constantly and she couldn't quiet him.

This went on for the first few weeks. He would scream in absolute terror. He wasn't in pain or hungry, just plain frightened. She held him to the light, but when he looked out the window he seemed to cry all the more. All that was out there was a range of beautiful mountains, one the legendary Superstition Mountain. Not knowing what else to do she put him down on the bed and said, "Son, I don't know what to do for you, I've done everything I can think of. If there's something bothering you, let me know somehow so I can help you."

She held him in her arms and looked deep into his eyes. He looked back in silent appeal, as though trying to make her understand. He had stopped crying for a moment, as if to convey something of his need. She went to sleep, praying the answer would come to her.

That night Sara had a dream. She dreamed she was watching a fight between Indian tribes and white soldiers on Superstition Mountain near Phoenix. The story went that one of the Indians, being pursued, lost his balance and fell end-over-end off a cliff to his death. In the dream the mother was standing where the body fell. She knew he had died yet, as she stood there, he got up and approached her, getting smaller with each step, until she recognized him as her newborn child.

The repeated turning from vertex to breech was almost a simulcast of the dream fall. Had the baby recalled a past life, in the womb, frightened even before he was born? The mother talked to him as she put him to sleep. She hugged and kissed him and looked deep into his eyes. He was no longer crying, as though he had surmised she had a message for him that would make everything all right. "You know, son," she said, "that was the last time. This time, Daddy and I are here to protect you. You don't need to worry or be frightened anymore."

She had a feeling he understood. It was the way he looked at her with unblinking eyes. When she said, "We love you. It's all over," his eyes drooped. He seemed relaxed. The frightened look was gone. He didn't scowl or scream and fell fast asleep in a matter of seconds. After that she had no more trouble with him. He was a happy normal baby. He no longer screamed, not even when he looked out the window at old Superstition Mountain.

It may have been a coincidence but the family soon left this mountain area and moved back to the great Northwest, where the mountains held no secret horrors nor the haunting tale of a death that wouldn't go away.

The Scarlet Letter

*On the breast of her gown,
in red cloth, appeared
the letter* A.

—Nathaniel Hawthorne
The Scarlet Letter

There was something about Rachel that was different. It wasn't her beauty, though she was beautiful, with her deep-set azure eyes and flowing blonde hair. There was something haunting about her face, as though it were from another time and place and bore a secret that no man knew. Yet she was dressed modishly with a skirt cut off at the knee and a low-cut blouse that revealed a patch of reddish skin. It looked like it could have been a birthmark, or an old lesion that hadn't healed.

It caught my eye. It looked like the capital letter **V**, two to three inches long and another inch or two wide, with an inside bar across. She was no more than 25, I decided. If she had worn a ruffled skirt and a white blouse to her neckline, she would have resembled one of the Puritan young women whose portraits adorn the Boston museums. There was an Old Worldliness about this young woman, a reserve. It was in the way she held her head and looked straight at you, then quickly averted her eyes as though afraid she may have appeared forward.

I saw no sign of illness in the pale features nor any uneasiness. "Why," I said with a smile, "have you come to me?"

The woman pointed to the mark on her chest, just below the collarbone. "This is why I am here. I want this red mark removed. It has plagued me long enough."

I leaned forward to more closely observe the reddish mark. "Have you seen anyone else about it?"

"Oh, yes, a dozen doctors—plastic surgeons, orthopedists, neural surgeons. Whatever. Nobody wants to touch it. They've never seen anything like it, and they're concerned that whatever they do will leave a scar. They said it's best to just keep it and and cover it with a blouse if it bothers me that much."

"That seems like sound advice," I said taking a second look. "It's really not that bad. Nobody would know it was there with a fuller blouse."

The young woman's lips met in a grim line. "I would. I think of it 24 hours a day. I can't get it out of my mind." She shook her head. "And I don't know why. That's the maddening part."

I was beginning to realize that I was dealing with something more than met the eye.

I reached out and touched the reddish skin. It was smooth under my touch, no scales, no ooziness or signs of infection. Whatever it was had completely healed.

"It looks harmless to me, somewhat like a birthmark. It's not like any scar I've seen. How did it happen?"

She hesitated a moment.

"I was wondering when you'd ask. It was quite a while ago, 10 years. I was 17 and a graduating senior in high school in Virginia. We were having a beach party. I was out in the sun all day, coming in and out of the water, surfing, swimming, having a good time. Being so fair, I got a terrible sunburn and I had chills all night. But in a week or so, the pain had disappeared, and so had the redness—except for this mark."

That in itself struck me as odd. Why would this capital **V** remain to bedevil this woman? And why did it disturb her so? Our eyes met across the desk.

"Is there anything else you can tell me? Any clue?"

"Not really." The young woman paused and a frown furrowed the lovely brow. "I have the strangest feeling at times that it all has happened before. But how could it have? I'm still not 30"— she laughed, and it was not a pretty laugh—"though I have lived enough for several lives."

The physician in me moved to the fore. "You really have nothing to worry about. There's no sign of malignancy or incipient tumor. Has it changed shape or color since it healed?"

"No, it remains the same."

"I suppose a plastic surgeon could remove it, if you wanted to bother, and graft some skin from elsewhere on your body."

"I don't want surgery." She paused. "I'm thinking of marrying. I want to come into that marriage with a whole skin and no memories from the past."

By this time I was fully aware that I was dealing with more an emotional problem than a physical one, one that might not so easily go away, even if the mark were removed. My office was jammed with patients, but how could I, a caring physician, let this troubled young woman go without first helping rouse the physician within her to assist in the deeper problem that was gnawing at her?

Rachel was frustrated, angered—even frightened—by this mark that had appeared out of thin air, so to speak, to become part of her every waking moment.

I was frankly mystified. "I don't know what to do about it, specifically," I said. "But I have two suggestions. One, you can put castor oil on it and see whether that tones down the skin somewhat. Secondly, you can concentrate on your dreams, asking them for help. Write them down as soon as you awake. When you come back in a month, we'll talk about it. Meanwhile, I'll do some thinking about that letter **V**. It must have some significance, to have taken the shape it has. It could very well be symbolic."

Rachel looked at me doubtfully. "Castor oil?"

I smiled. "Just dream away. We'll go on from there. You mentioned something about a feeling it had all happened before. Did you visualize anything? A face, a place, a time?"

Rachel shook her head. "That was what was so strange. I kept seeing my own face, and I seemed to be sobbing, always sobbing."

"And this happened when the mark appeared?"

"Yes, along with a good many other things, which I don't like getting into."

I held back a sigh. "As you will. We'll talk it through when you come back and see if we can come to some resolution. Just jot down your dreams the first thing in the morning. I'll do some thinking about it as well. I have a hunch we'll come up with something."

I had a feeling Rachel would be back. And she was. One month to the day.

She hadn't used the castor oil, but she had recorded her dreams. They were all in black and white: a nun in a black habit and a bride in a white dress; a black cat and a white cat. There was no other color. I could see Rachel was even more interested now to solve this little mystery. There is nothing more intriguing than a mystery, especially when it revolves around ourselves. I gave the red patch of skin a cursory glance. It hadn't changed and I hadn't expected it to—not until this puzzle was solved.

Rachel was sitting in a comfortable chair, looking at me with those blue eyes that held mine like a vise. Not wanting to beat about the bush I said, "Now, as you grew up, was everything black and white in your life? Was everything either right or it was wrong, with no gray areas?"

Rachel nodded. "Yes. In my church, there were no two ways about anything. Everything was either black or white, right or wrong, and usually it was wrong."

I smiled. "Because you made it wrong?"

"In some ways," she replied.

Rachel was perfectly at ease. It was as if she had finally worked something out in her mind. Had the dreams touched a forgotten chord?

"Okay," I said, "now we're getting somewhere. You had something to conform to—right and wrong—something that was a solid part of your life. When this mark appeared after the beach party, was there anything else going on in your life? Something to do with black and white, right and wrong?"

"Well, I had this bad sunburn, as I said, starting with that beach party." She hesitated, then sighed. "I might as well get it out. Some of us began doing drugs and fooling around, just for kicks. I got into sex when I shouldn't have, and into drinking. I'd never had a drink before. That was a wrong thing. And I became pregnant. I couldn't tell my family because they would have disowned me. They were strict, rigid Catholics. I had an abortion without their knowing about it. Everything was piling up and I felt so guilty. But I was into it too deeply to stop. I felt I was killing something and this was against everything my family and my church stood for, and I even felt that way myself. But what was I to do? It would have hurt everybody if I had gone ahead and had the baby. It would have been the end of everything."

This, as I saw it, was a plea for understanding and forgiveness. This need for forgiveness had something to do with the red mark on her chest. If she got rid of the mark, the need for forgiveness might go. Now she had exculpated herself—or had she? There was more, much more to tell, and it flowed out of all the soul-searching.

For the next few years, Rachel told me, she drifted aimlessly. She would take a job as a waitress every now and then, and she moved from one boyfriend to another, getting deeper into the quagmire of self-pity and guilt, knowing intuitively, without knowing how, that the red mark on her chest was her badge of shame.

I was trying to put everything in place. As I kept scrutinizing the V-shaped reddish patch, I realized that the V upside down, with the inside bar, was a perfect capital A. I was excited. I knew what this meant. But kids today didn't read the old classics. I turned from that thought for a moment, intending to get back to it when the conversation permitted. The depth of Rachel's guilt was heavy enough to weigh anyone down. Hopefully, the marriage would help turn that around. So, too, would a return to Christ and a Christ-consciousness. That was what Christ was all about: love and forgiveness. Without this, the best doctor—or preacher—couldn't heal anyone.

I took the girl's hand and squeezed it. I wanted her to know that I understood and that I would do all I could to awaken the physician within her and let her know she didn't stand alone.

"You have to put some of the past behind you. You will go on and have other children, and that will make up for some of it. It was a learning experience. Don't be too hard on yourself."

Rachel winced. "It is a mortal sin in the church's eyes. And in mine. No matter what I tell myself."

"And you wholly believe this?"

"Yes, from childhood. Why wouldn't I? But you can't go around having babies you can't take care of. I felt guilty about what I did, going along with the abortion, but I couldn't marry; I was only a teenager." Tears came to her eyes. "It was awful. Real bad. At one time I felt there was no way out."

I took another look at the V-shaped lesion with a little bar across it. A perfect A, if inverted. A, the Scarlet Letter. A for Adultery, a stigma in old Salem that would never die.

"Did you ever read *The Scarlet Letter* by Nathaniel Hawthorne?"

Rachel nodded. "I wondered when you were coming to that. Yes, in our senior year, just before graduation. It was a class assignment. I guess they were trying to knock something into my head."

"Then you read it around the time of the picnic, the one where you kids sort of let go?"

"You could put it that way."

"And it all came tumbling down on you at once?"

"Yes, it was real bad. I got tired of feeling guilty. I tried to justify myself, but I couldn't do it."

"You were familiar with the name Hester Prynne."

"Oh, yes, I can hardly forget her. She reminded me so much of myself. With the letter A for Adulteress. She was the one they put on a scaffold in the town market so everyone could witness her shame."

So she was familiar with the character of Hester Prynne, the young woman who had a baby by a lover who betrayed her, leaving her to the mercies of the Salem witchcraft mob.

Rachel blushed and went on. "I sympathized with her, especially when I became pregnant. I wondered what she would have thought. I could picture how she looked. I saw her as pretty much like me. When I read where they put her up on a scaffold in the town square and mocked her, I wanted to cry. Then they put her in jail and there was nobody to help her. The last humiliation came when they sewed the scarlet letter **A** into the embroidery of her dress."

I empathized with the young woman who had suffered so much for what she had done to herself, knowing she was doing wrong, committing a mortal sin, compounded by the abortion which had rent her soul with guilt.

Why was this girl so driven? Why this red letter, symbolic of Adulteress? And why had she come to me? Then it hit me. I was the one doctor who made no secret of my belief in the continuity of life, in reincarnation. I had been ridiculed by conventional religionists who blocked out the many references to reincarnation in the Bible. I decided I wouldn't mince words with this candid young woman who had dug so deeply into herself.

"Did you by any chance recall anything of that time in Salem, besides what you may have read?"

Rachel's eyes widened. "I sometimes thought I saw a small square, with the men dressed in knickers and stockings, the women in frilly dresses. But it could have been my imagination. I vaguely saw the face of a young woman who looked like me, I thought. But that, too, could have been my wandering mind. I had a feeling of intense distaste for everything I saw in the town square. In the end, I decided, it all was a dream, a bad dream."

She shook her head, and her eyes had a mournful look. "That's what I kept telling myself when I was going through all that business of being shuttled around after the abortion: This is a bad dream. But it hurt too much for a dream."

I thought about it. When would the hurt end? And when would its painful reminder go away, the red inverted **V** that prolonged that hurt? She had come almost full circle, but not quite. She was seeking what that other woman, Hester Prynne, had not found: a great peace within her, and redemption—the same redemption that Hester Prynne had been denied. Hester Prynne had loved the man she was pregnant by and had kept the baby. The Hester Prynne character had a strength Rachel lacked, and her guilt was perhaps not as great, because she had loved without being promiscuous. The person who truly loves is the gainer. Her soul is clearer. She has not sinned in her own light.

My mind went over what I knew of the book and the gifted author. A transcendentalist like Thoreau and Emerson, Hawthorne humanized his fictional character. But how fictional were they? Hawthorne wrote frequently of what he actually experienced, transforming his experienced to suit a novelist's fancy. There were many Hester Prynnes in colonial Salem and other dark corners of the Massachusetts Bay Colony, and they paid dearly for any moment of weakness and forbidden love. Hester's sin was more heinous than even a witch's in old Salem, and she had been memorialized down the years in plays and movies until she became the prototype of a fallen woman.

Had Rachel thought she was any of these poor creatures? The idea passed through my mind. The inverted **A** appeared on Rachel's chest when she was suffering bitter pangs of guilt from her sexual lapses and an abortion. All this happened while she had been compelled in school to read about the downfall of a young woman to whom it was all too easy to relate.

As I looked across my desk, I couldn't help thinking how this girl might have suffered in another time, with every act of vilification that had been heaped on Hester.

Had she indeed empathized with Hawthorne's scarlet lady?

Rachel lowered her eyes. "It would have been hard not to. That image of her never left me. I wept until there were no longer tears in my eyes."

Without playing psychiatrist, I ran this scenario through my mind. The subconscious mind, so intimately connected with every cell in the body, may very well have produced this badge of guilt on poor Rachel's body where it was plainly visible. Her guilt feeling was so great that she had been flagellating herself all this time. Now, with a marriage in sight, hopefully she was approaching the end of her ordeal, something that had been denied Hester Prynne.

The inverted **A** was still a puzzle. Why had the scarlet letter labeling the girl's shame manifested itself upside down?

I thought about it. Hester Prynne was condemned by the narrow-minded townspeople of Salem, but Rachel was putting the label on herself. It was a self-inflicted wound, the complete reverse—upside down. Her subconscious mind saw it that way. The feeling was so strong, to the depths of her very soul, that it sent a message to the innate intelligence of every cell in her body—and the result was the mark on her chest. This was why she didn't conceal it. It was part of her punishment.

The question now was, how could she be helped to enter into her marriage with a clear head and a clear heart? How could she turn all this guilt around and heal herself? Where would she find the physician within to help her?

We talked about that. Rachel had gone against her principles, but she was basically a good person, still wedded to her early beliefs. Without those beliefs, she wouldn't have suffered as she had. Now it was time she understood that we don't forgive ourselves, God forgives us. I pointed out that Jesus' approach to people who strayed was not to condemn them but to help them bring forgiveness into their lives, and to accept that forgiveness. We're the ones who reject forgiveness. Forgiveness is always there, like the air that's around us all the time. We're the ones who stop breathing. Rachel was caught up in condemnation in her own consciousness. This consciousness had to be replaced by a true Christ-consciousness. Christ always forgave, even at the cross.

We talked about the little red mark, the "brand" that said so much, and when Rachel left, she was already feeling better about herself. As planned, she married and soon had a child. It was my feeling that the brand would go away by itself now that Rachel had someone of her own to love. Love and forgiveness go together. There was no balm in Gilead, nor in old Salem. But I had an idea Rachel would find it in the here and now. With all her soul-stirring, she had found the physician within.

Listening to the Voice of Illness

It is not all life to live.
Nor yet all of death to die.

—EDGAR CAYCE

Can illness be our friend? It can be, when it is a way of contacting the physician within. I have a friend who says illness is social communication. It's a way that the body has of saying both to us and to the world around us, "Hey gang, there's really something wrong here. Will you please do something about it?"

So many of us ignore the symptoms of illness until we're really sick. We're often afraid those symptoms may represent something we don't want to know about, and if we don't pay attention to them, they will go away. Because of our ideology of accountability, we tend to think of illness as punishment, something we must endure. But illness is the body saying "pay attention, help me." We need to listen to our bodies, to the physician within who so often speaks indirectly to us.

I did just that in a recent case. An attractive woman in her 30s came to our Scottsdale clinic not for herself, but for her sick father. He turned out not to be very sick at all, suffering a mild gastritis, and craving attention. My attention turned to the daughter, the goodwill messenger. She seemed distracted, nervous, with an unhealthy pallor and deep circles under her eyes. She was obviously not sleeping well, and she was preoccupied to the extent that she didn't appear to notice anyone, even when addressed directly. I decided that of the two, the daughter had a more urgent need, but how was I to get her attention? She was very much into herself.

She was sitting across the desk from me discussing her father's illness when a thought occurred to me and I said, "Have you had any bad dreams lately?"

She looked up, startled. The question seemed to have come out of nowhere. She hesitated and then heaved a big sigh. "I don't know how you got that, but the last two years have been a nightmare. I don't sleep very well, and when I do, I dream the same dream over and over, and it always wakes me up. Then I can't fall back to sleep."

She drew her hand across her face, and her eyes closed for a moment. "This dream never leaves me. It takes over at any time. I have no power over it."

I saw the lines in the still youthful face and I saw the tremor in her hands. She was obviously suffering from chronic fatigue and getting by on nerve alone, making herself ill. Soon she would run out of reserves, with the predictable result.

Whatever she had been living with was so disturbing that it was a struggle to get it out. She finally came to a decision. There is something about listening, keeping focused and showing interest that opens people's hearts.

"Yes," she said, "it might be better if I did talk about it. I didn't want to get into any psychiatry. I'm not crazy. I'm angry, desperate. I don't want to change. I'll never change." Her eyes flared for a moment, then she leaned back in her chair, emotionally spent.

"I don't know how I can help," I said evenly. "But it might be a good idea to get the anger out and take a look at it in the daylight. It's amazing how much it helps to see things in the light."

The woman frowned. "That may have been why I came here with my dad. He could have come alone. Maybe it was something I needed to do. And this was the time."

I reached out and touched her hand. "Just tell me what you like, stopping whenever you feel like it."

Once she made up her mind, turbulent as it was, there was no holding back. The anger and frustration gushed out of her like a river bursting a dam and splashing downstream. And it was no wonder. The story was appalling.

"Four years ago I discovered my husband sexually molesting our two small boys. I was horrified. I went to the authorities. There was a trial and he was jailed, but the term wasn't long enough. No term could have been. I took care of the boys for two years, loving them and worrying what would happen when he got out. I asked the prison officials, the probation department and others to let me know when he was being released. I knew his getting sent away for so brief a period would not be enough to stop him. First, he would try to get back at me. Then he would try to get the boys again, to do what he wanted with them. I shuddered when I thought about it. My bad dreams began."

The words rolled out of her like a breaking storm. She kept asking about his release and nobody could give her a date. "They couldn't care less. He was paroled without my knowing about it. Then the worst happened. Every weekday I drove the boys to school and told them I'd be picking them up later. One afternoon I drove to the school at closing time and was told they had already been picked up—by their father. The words sent a chill through me. All kinds of thoughts whirled through my mind, all of them too horrible to contemplate."

She reported the kidnapping, but the man and the two children seemed to have disappeared off the face of the earth. He could have taken them overseas, anywhere. There was no trace. She had spent the last two years searching, grasping at every clue. She didn't know if her children were dead or alive. She was driven by her love for them and her fierce hatred for their father. And every night she had the same dream. It had taken over her life.

In this dream, she saw herself walking into the kitchen, there encountering her husband fondling her two boys. She became furious, picking up a knife and lunging at him. Each time she did this he would grab one of the children, throw him up as a shield, and she would stab one of the boys instead. With a cry of horror, shivering, she would wake up with the sensation of warm blood, the blood of her children, on her hands. She found it impossible to get back to sleep. The dream never varied. This went on for two years. The strain, the loss of sleep, the imagery, the uncertainty about the children's whereabouts and welfare ate away at her. She was a nervous wreck, all the more so because she held it all in.

There was a message in her dream, but she wasn't getting it. The message was obvious, but she was too involved to see it, too angry. Her dream was actually the physician within her, her subconscious mind, trying to save her from herself and the terrible anger consuming her. I pointed out that her subconscious was telling her very clearly, with graphic reality, that her anger wasn't hurting the target—her husband—but the children she loved. It couldn't have been plainer.

She heard me out. But she had held this anger for so long she still wasn't ready to release it. "How can I forgive him," she asked, "when I think about what he may be doing this very moment." Her lips curled in disgust.

"I can see where that would be difficult," I said. "But rather than putting all your energy into hating him, which does you no good, why not transpose that same energy into love and send it to your children wherever they are. It will reach them. Love accomplishes wonders."

"You mean they will know that I'm thinking of them and that I love them?"

"I'm sure of that. And say a little prayer for them, too. And put all your energy into it. They will know it, and think of you. And you will see how much better you feel."

It did do some good. She banished her husband from her thoughts that night and concentrated on her children. She saw them in the kitchen of a nondescript home, and they were all right. This was a very clear impression. She slept through the night, awakening invigorated and optimistic. She was no longer in malaise, no longer beset with pain generated by feelings of anguish and hopelessness. She told herself that some day those children would be back, unscathed.

She had been on the verge of a breakdown without knowing it. But in blocking off the hatred and anger, she opened her sub-conscious mind and got in touch with the depth of pain she needed to work through. It turned her around emotionally, a wonder accomplished by love.

And the children? This is an unfinished story. But whenever they come back, and she believes they will now, her heart will be full of love for them, not heavy with rancor and resentment. The pain left her, and she is ready to go on. Perhaps not to forgive, but to go on.

How do we awaken the physician within? What do we do? What techniques do we have? As a doctor, one of the most helpful things I can do is encourage my patients to be in touch with their own body, to really feel it. Does it feel sound and firm, healthy and aware?

Women are very touchy about their breasts. Healthwise, it is one of the most significant female organs. The concept of breast examinations is extremely important and has saved many lives. With the medical profession's overemphasis on the vulnerability of a woman's breasts, however, we may have inadvertently created a lot of masses in that area. I tell my women patients to examine their breasts every month, but not to be obsessed with lumps. If a woman thinks she will find lumps, she may get lumps, because the thought has already formed in the subconscious mind. It's like pain. Almost any part of your body will hurt if you think pain there long enough.

When women do their monthly breast exams, they should do so with a light thought, "Hello, girls, how are you today? What is going on? Do you have a message for me?" Women should not check with fear, but respect that their bodies will let them know what's going on. As with the rest of the body, women should give their breasts the care and attention they need.

My patients often call on their physician within when I'm not available. One patient of mine had gone to a specialist in nearby Flagstaff. She questioned his diagnosis of a urinary tract infection. She called me late in the day on a Friday to discuss the situation, but I missed her call. I knew she would get back to me if she had to.

Later, she told me that the more she had thought about it, the more sure she was that the diagnosis was wrong. As she had before when ill, she started to meditate, sinking into her subconscious level. She heard a small voice saying with unmistakable emphasis, "It is not a urinary infection. It's a yeast infection."

The following morning she went back to the local doctor and told him what the physician within had said—without giving that physician a name or an address.

The doctor bridled a little. "How do you know?"

"I just know," she said, as though not wishing to betray a confidence.

The physician had more tests done. It turned out that the little voice within was right. The doctor treated her accordingly. By the time I called her Monday morning she was feeling so much better she was no longer annoyed with me for not calling her back.

In another intriguing case, I had a young woman patient, an expectant mother, who had kidney problems. She was more than six months' pregnant, and I thought she should be having a lot of pain from the pressure of the fetus on the kidneys. She would come into the office and I would say, "Kathy, are you having much pain?" And she would say no. This happened a couple of times and finally I said, "Why aren't you having pain? You should be having pain."

Kathy hesitated a moment, then smiled. "I guess," she said, "I learned from my physician within how to detach my mind. At the first twinge of pain I leave my body, escaping the pain."

I shook my head. She had learned only too well. "I don't think that's a really good idea," I said, "because now is the time when your baby needs you in your body, while it is developing."

When it was time for Kathy to deliver, she had a difficult labor, a breech delivery. Every so often in the midst of this labor, she would lift her head and say with a wan smile, "Well, Doctor Gladys, I'm still in my body." The nurses didn't know what she was talking about and thought she was out of her mind. But we knew what was going on. And the baby, a healthy specimen, was delivered without any further problem.

I frequently utilize the physician within a patient when there's confusion about diagnosis and treatment, particularly with infants who are not old enough to speak intelligibly and who can only cry when the pain becomes severe. One little patient of mine, a beautiful 18-month-old baby girl with golden curls and big blue eyes, looked up at her elders with a light in her baby face. Then one day her smile and laughter turned to tears. The first indication of a problem came when her parents found blood and mucous in her diapers. They took her from doctor to doctor trying to find someone who could help her, or even make a diagnosis. "My own fear fell like a sledge hammer," the grandmother said, "the day my daughter asked the city's most prominent pediatrician if she should take the baby to Children's Hospital, and he shook his head.

"'No,' he said, 'just keep doing what you're doing. Maybe she'll outgrow it.'

"We knew only too well what that meant," the grandmother went on to say. "They didn't know what the problem was and they didn't want the responsibility."

Meanwhile the young mother kept rummaging though health and medical journals and books, searching for a clue to the child's condition and what could be done about it. The little girl was always hungry but could tolerate only a few foods. She was increasingly cranky, wanting to be held all the time. Her family took her to the hospital for tests, and vials of blood were taken from this anemic child. The grandmother went along with the mother. She recalled: "The doctor prescribed liquid iron. As soon as we gave her the prescribed dose it would shoot out of her mouth. I asked the doctor if there was a better way to give her the iron. He said no, and that we must give it to her. Her hemoglobin seemed to be getting slightly higher but she seemed to be getting worse. She was so weak and cranky, she could barely lift a hand.

"The baby was admitted to the hospital's gastrointestinal department in a room with three other children. I mentioned to the chief doctor that their hematology department was using liquid iron for the child. 'Oh,' he smiled, 'we don't use that. It's too hard on their colons. I don't think they assimilate iron in that form.'"

There was also difficulty with the hospital diet. The mother had been selecting all the cooked fresh vegetables she could find on the hospital's menus. One day she objected to the fried chicken nuggets they were about to feed her child. She was chided by the doctor. "Don't pressure the other doctors about diet. There's a law in this state. The doctors can invoke this law at any time and use any treatment they choose."

The grandmother could hardly believe what she'd heard. "Is this," she thought, "the dark age of medicine?"

After numerous tests, the doctors advised the parents that the child had Crohn's disease. The mother was relieved to have a diagnosis, but her relief was short-lived. One doctor briefed her: "The only thing that's worse is liver failure." Another said, "Leukemia is better. At least we can cure leukemia."

The doctors explained that with Crohn's disease the colon becomes inflamed. Blood and mucous form. The disease was chronic. They didn't know the cause and there was no cure.

"The best they could do," said the grandmother, "was to treat the child with prednisone, a steroid. They said she would be on this medication the rest of her life, however long that was. After a few treatments she developed the puffed cheeks, glassy eyes, and skinny arms and legs of someone on prednisone."

At this point the mother, hearing about our clinic, decided to call me in Scottsdale. She described the symptoms, the diagnosis and the treatment. I nodded at the other end of the line and suggested she read a book called *The Yeast Connection*. I had an idea from what she said that a yeast infection could very well be the problem, and not incurable Crohn's disease. The symptoms were often similar. There was a way of making sure. "Give her some plain yogurt every day—not much, just a spoonful or two."

The doctors demurred, but the yogurt seemed to help. The child became calmer, less cranky.

As soon as the child was stronger so that the family could fly across country with her, I agreed to take her as a patient.

The day after the baby left the hospital, the grandmother and mother, with the child and her three-year-old brother piled in their laps, took the last two seats on a plane for Phoenix-Scottsdale. They were greeted by the clinic staff and myself with a hug and a smile. They stayed for a month in a motel room. I tested the child and her mother and they both were loaded with candida (yeast), with no beneficial bacteria present. There was no incurable Crohn's disease. I prescribed a drug, Nystatin, for the mother, and a new diet for the child—only the freshest cooked food, especially vegetables, together with freshly squeezed fruit juice, plain yogurt and no sugar or bleached flour—and nothing with yeast.

The child was soon vastly improved. The little family, home-sick after a month, flew back East to rejoin the child's father. There was a minor setback. "Without the steadfast care of Dr. Gladys," said the grandmother, "the symptoms came back and the child was rushed to the hospital. She was put on intravenous fluids and allowed no food by mouth. Her bowel blew up with toxins and could have burst."

In a panic, the mother called me in Scottsdale. "Tell your doctors to give the little girl some yogurt at once," I said.

The chief doctor agreed. He prescribed a spoonful of yogurt three times a day, even though he still didn't believe the disease was yeast connected. The child responded immediately, her colon becoming normal.

"Today, two years later," the grandmother reports, "she is a beautiful healthy child. She was gradually weaned off the prednisone and lost her puffy cheeks. The scar on her chest from the intravenous connection to her heart is barely visible. Her bones are still brittle and thin from her brief stint on the steroid, but the muscles on her legs, arms and body are firm and well-toned. She is a healthy, happy child. I'm full of joy at her complete recovery. I thank God to whom I prayed so often. I thank the mother, my daughter, for her steadfast courage in the face of great medical opposition. And I thank Dr. McGarey for combining regular medicine and holistic medicine to give our wonderful child a real cure."

I was pleased but ready to share the accolades with the mother and grandma, and with the remarkable physician within each of them helping the child they loved.

A Matter of Faith

*I can do all things through Christ
who strengthens me.*

— Philippians 4:13

They spoke of support groups—people in the same boat as them, sitting around and discussing their illnesses, and getting what support they could out of the others' experiences. It was heartening for some. But for Ruth Bydon there could be no such sessions. Not when she was so allergic to an attending doctor's suit of clothes, recently dry-cleaned, that he was compelled to change his suit or lose a patient.

Ruth had the greatest conglomeration of allergies that I, as a doctor, had ever encountered. This meant, of course, that she had a deficient immune system. She was almost isolated, screened from visitors who could endanger her life by their presence. I visited her only when it was absolutely necessary and I was sure, after some self-examination, that I was nontoxic. Her case was so unusual, not only from the rarity of her symptomatic picture, but for the problem it presented for others, especially her husband. He needed the patience and endurance of Job, but he was invariably upbeat, and that helped both of them.

Knowing the isolation in which she lived, I called ahead one day, inquiring whether I might bring a reporter friend interested in the human drama surrounding Ruth's very special case. He was told what he could and couldn't wear, but even with that, there was still some uneasiness on Ruth's part about the visit. We stopped by in the later afternoon when her husband would be home to share the burden of receiving a stranger.

The reporter was quite adaptable, not minding being gone over with a fine comb before he was permitted to enter the modest Bydon home. Fortunately, he didn't smoke or drink, as even a hint of nicotine or alcohol could touch off a nasty asthmatic attack. Our clothes had to be of natural fabric, no polyester or the like. We deposited our shoes at the door. Happily, the reporter didn't use cologne, any scent or harsh soaps.

We looked around the tidy living room. No rugs or drapes. They picked up contaminants. The floors were clean and the wood chairs and tables free of dust. Ruth and her husband Gary looked like any normal youngish couple, attractive, relaxed, interested. As a minister, Gary was totally committed to Ruth's support. Helping her had deepened his faith and made it highly personal. He had become patient, flexible and practical, even to keeping a set of dry-cleaned clothes at the church, which he never brought home.

As usual his eyes were fixed on his wife, anticipating her least want, deferring to her when she spoke. It could not have been easy, commuting from his Nevada church to the three or four cities where she had been hospitalized as doctors puzzled over a variety of ailments which induced a subnormal immune system. As we spoke Ruth kept breathing in oxygen from a tube to control her asthma. She had other ailments: arthritis, osteoporosis, vasculitis. She had been a preemie baby, one of twins. It was thought that her immune system hadn't developed sufficiently in the fetal stage to ward off the countless allergens in the air, food and water. Having been a nurse for a good many years, Ruth took care of herself until her abnormal sensitivity to the environment got to be too much for her. There were early indications of severe allergy problems, but a serious lapse, making her an invalid, didn't occur until 1984. In 1994 she came to our clinic in Scottsdale, and began a daily regimen following a stringent diet and visualizing her wellness. After two years, she began to perk up, doing her own housework and looking forward to a career of helping people, sharing her unique experience as a patient who had been given so much.

There were discouraging moments, but with Gary's help and the substantial participation of an active congregation and their prayers, we were making the transition back to health and well-being.

There was no doubt in Gary's mind that the prayers and the help of the congregation had pulled them through. It hadn't been easy. "The power of prayer, individually and collectively, had a lot to do with Ruth's improvement," Gary made clear.

When a variety of treatments elsewhere for her asthmatic attacks had failed, Gary brought her to the Scottsdale area. He took her first to a local doctor known for her expertise in diagnosis. After examining Ruth she took Gary into another room and said:

"Mr. Bydon, your wife could stop breathing at any moment. Her throat is blue. I can't give her any more steroids, any more benadryl, or her heart may stop."

A shiver went through Gary. "Doctor, do you have any recommendations?"

She shook her head. "None. I can't treat her anymore because
she's reached the limit of the medications we can give under
standard medical practice, and I have no recommendations at
this particular time. Good luck."

After that, there came desperate visits to Chicago and Dallas
hospitals, with Gary commuting from Nevada every two or three
weeks after his wife was hospitalized. Science, focusing on a
disease that few understood instead of on the whole person,
had failed.

There were times when both Ruth and Gary were weary and
depressed. Ruth thought she was being punished for the twin
who had died when she was born, and Gary tried to play it
down. He had something going for himself and his wife of 20
years. He was a minister, and ministers, like the religion they
espoused, were called on to succor the sick and the lame and
not ask why.

Gary looked now at his wife, still beautiful with an inner
glow, and love tempered his voice.

"It wasn't easy coming into this world for Ruth. When I first
met her we were in junior high. She was barely a teenager and
already asthmatic. She was taking all kinds of medication:
steroids, bronchial dilators, painkillers. The doctors told her she
would grow out of it, and there were periods of remission. But
not many."

They were married when he was in the seminary. They came
to Nevada because of the dryness of the climate—fewer pollutants, fewer pollens, more space.

Both felt it would take a Higher Power to see them through.
"Being a minister helped and hindered. I was expected to have
all the answers, connections and insight. I didn't. In so many
hard spots I was like everyone else, not knowing every twist or

turn of God's purpose. It made me humble, it turned my thinking around, making my humility a badge of honor. If God called
me to be a minister, I decided there must be a purpose in all
this suffering. We are only given so much to see. The rest is
invested in our faith. We are part of a larger spiritual universe
than we can imagine. What happens to each of us often has a
larger component than we are able to understand without
divine help. That component involves the role of the battle
between good and evil, a struggle I am just beginning to grasp.
It begins within each of us, and it ends with us. We each tune
into a universe which has been made ready for us by men of
clear vision given them by the Lord."

Through much of this conversation Ruth had been sitting quietly, breathing in occasionally on her oxygen tube. She smiled
now, in good spirits, obviously mending. "I prayed a lot," she
said. "I was always praying. That's why I've improved so much.
I think God's sick and tired of hearing my prayers."

Before Ruth got involved with the Scottsdale Holistic Medical
Group, the asthmatic attacks had become progressively harder
and more frequent. She wasn't digesting her food, and she
became exhausted quickly. She lost her hair and her weight got
down to 87 pounds. She was suffering from something new, the
malabsorption syndrome, and though she ate wholesome foods,
her body wouldn't digest or assimilate them. She was nothing
but skin and bone.

"We were still looking for doctors who could help," Gary said.
"Once we had to fly her to San Diego by air ambulance, with a
doctor and two nurses aboard. If we'd gone by car she would
have been exposed to exhaust fumes. Then she was flown in an
air ambulance from San Diego to Dallas, to a specialist who ran
an environmental control unit. Meanwhile, I was building a house
to fit the medical specifications of her environmentalist doctor."

The reporter's head came up. "Medical specifications?"

"Yes, this Nevada house we live in now. Everything is designed to accommodate Ruth's allergies: a porcelain enamel bedroom; three different air systems; an air-conditioning unit and filtration system for the main part of the house; heat pumps for different rooms; a clean room with its own heat pump. There's no paint in the house, and the plaster doesn't have lye in it."

Ruth's complex disorder, I had explained, involved the breakdown of her weakest parts and organs when her immune system was at its lowest point. Her psyche, her mental and emotional side, was involved with the physical and beyond the scope of specialists concerned only with their specialties.

The twin who died when Ruth was born had always been a problem of the spirit. All her life she had worked to separate herself from this twin and from the guilt of her being stillborn, strangled by Ruth's umbilical cord. Ruth couldn't accept this death. She had a need to bring this twin into the light, beginning to realize that in her guilt over the twin's death she had a suppressed wish to join her. She began to understand this through her visualizations and meditations in this inner world of hers. Finally, she came to know that she had to release the dead twin to stay alive in the real world.

"As I released control a Higher Power brought down the wall in my life, a wall that I rarely spoke of or acknowledged. I was no longer in need of my twin's help. I finally saw the unreality was my own. My purpose now was clear—to help others through life's journey. Through my suffering, others may come closer to the universal power. I can help those who are ill by setting an example, getting myself better and not giving in."

Gary's Nevada church had made itself a major support group. "There was a constancy in their support and love that gave me the strength I had asked of God. I didn't have to look far to find the Lord. I saw his presence in every face in my congregation."

Despite her illness and near brushes with death, Ruth retained her optimism in the healing process. Her weight had increased from the meager 87 pounds to a normal 110. Her vitality had noticeably increased. She spoke with animation and humor, with lightheartedness. She was able to laugh at herself, something that I, her present physician, considered one of the basic ingredients of any true healing.

"There was a joke around," Ruth smiled, "that I was getting better because God was tired of hearing about me from so many people."

Gary, working with his own physician within, had found himself becoming something of a diagnostician. "Necessity, they say, is the mother of invention. You never know when the necessity may arise. The least thing could touch off an attack in Ruth's autoimmune complex, with the body reacting against itself violently. In the first week at the Chicago hospital, we almost lost her to severe asthma attacks. Every time the doctor would come in to treat her in protective isolation, Ruth would have a severe allergic attack. The doctor was contemplating bringing in a psychiatrist. Obviously, there was something about him she was reacting to. But it wasn't in her mind. He had on a freshly dry-cleaned suit, and that was doing it—the dry-cleaning fluid."

Ruth found herself playing nurse. But there was only so much she could do. "In the beginning I had more of a focus on the medical part. What I had was undefined in medical terms. There was this vasculitis, a breakdown within the blood vessels. I worked in intensive care as a nurse for many years, so I looked at what was going on in a medical way. But I knew nothing about vasculitis. I was frustrated and upset with the separations and setbacks. But there was nothing we could do but stay together. We had married for a reason. That reason hadn't changed—to live together in love for the rest of our days."

A smile flit across her face. "People say, 'I don't see how you can go through all this.' I don't look at it that way. I take it one day at a time. I'm improving rapidly with Dr. Gladys. I'm even enjoying doing housework again."

Gary found that Ruth's outbreaks of different diseases varied with her immune system. "She's had considerable pain. She takes injectable benadryl for the allergies, and painkilling drugs. The blood vessel problem, the vasculitis, appeared in the last two or three years. If anyone walks into the house with a strong cologne on you can see her legs turn blue. The circulation to the lower extremities bogs down on allergic exposure.

"Meanwhile," he bowed in my direction, "Gladys has been bringing Ruth to a point now where she is comfortable with herself. Always supportive of Ruth's inner sense of what needed to be done, Gladys established an instant rapport with Ruth. She's a rare physician who doesn't get in the way of the physician within the patient. Gladys works with the patient, through visualization and meditation, to allow the healing to work within."

Ruth hadn't done any housework in years, but it was more than doing housework now. It was getting back to normalcy, and doing something for Gary who had done so much for her. "Sometimes," said Gary, "maids created more problems with the pollutants they'd bring in than anything they could do helping Ruth. We were running out of people who could clean the house, and out of necessity Ruth started doing a little more. And I helped out.

"All this was happening at once. I don't think it would have happened without the new confidence that came with Gladys and her upbeat team. Not only did Ruth feel physically supported, but spiritually and psychologically comfortable. In a new comfort zone, with confidence, she could reach out a little further."

Ruth expanded on this. "That doesn't mean I didn't have a day or two where I didn't want to just throw something or be angry and cry and be all upset. But I've decided healing is not just for the patient but for those around her. When I first started getting sick, we worked with a pastor friend of Gary. He got upset with Gary and with me. 'Why is she so sick all the time?' he'd say. 'What's going on here? Why don't you send her to a psychiatrist?' He wasn't much help, but he did hang on for a while, not believing anyone could be sick all the time like I was without dying.

"Then some years later his daughter fell ill. It was a difficult illness, hard to treat. She had developed endometriosis, which was difficult to pinpoint and treat. Part of the uterine lining breaks off and goes up the fallopian tubes and into the abdominal cavity. Every time the poor girl had her period there was bleeding in her abdomen. With her illness, he became more understanding of mine. He said that without the relationship we had had, and what he and his wife saw us go through, they could never have given their daughter the support they did. This made me feel my sickness had served some purpose."

Ruth had looked so well that the doctors thought it was all in her head. "No matter how sick she was, she took pride in her personal appearance," Gary recalled. "Until she went into a complete relapse and lost that 25 pounds."

They had operated to remove blood clots formed by allergic deposits in her bloodstream. The surgeons took a look at her vena cava, the blood vessel returning the blood to the heart, and said it was only by the grace of God that she was still alive. If one of those blood clots had moved it would have been instant death.

"It was at this point that we decided we needed a physician who was more open, who would listen, who would look at all of Ruth, not just a leg or an arm—someone who would view her as a friend, a person."

Our conversation had gone all around the clock. I could see at this point that the reporter was wondering what had turned

Ruth around. So much had been done for her, and to her, that it was difficult to put a finger on what altered her course. All the prayer in the world wouldn't do that unless the patient's motivation goal were clearly focused. With Ruth's having been a nurse for several years, I had the feeling that her physician within had told her that the route she was taking could have only one conclusion: death. She had to dig in and take an active role in her own healing. Ruth had much to live for—her husband, their friends and her growing awareness, through exposure to so much medical care, of the widespread failure of conventional medicine to tap into the individual. It occurred to her that having been a nurse *and* a patient, she could be of benefit to others if she drew herself out of the mire of her illness. Then she could proclaim, "If I did it, so can you." It was at this point that Ruth came to our clinic, and holistically, things began to move into place.

"I did the biofeedback and the visualization with the psychologist. I received acupuncture to relieve the pain. Finally, the therapeutic massage put me in touch with my body. It was very much alive. Conventional medicines had almost killed me twice, so I welcomed the visualization program with the biofeedback."

As her physician, I watched Ruth's horizons expand and I had the feeling that she was ready for a comeback. One of her dreams had been to have a child, but she's a very practical person and she realized that her dream of bearing a child was just that: a dream. She was now 40 and under the best of circumstances there might have been problems with a firstborn. She had a new and spiritually motivated purpose—to help people, to serve as an example for the sick who had lost hope. To do that she had to get well and behave like a well person. She wanted to become active again, and hoped to eventually get back into nursing. She was particularly good at visualization, and Gary had trained at an Eastern pain-control center to reinforce images for Ruth. For example, she couldn't take any medication for pain. So the first thing Gary did when she came out of surgery was to touch her wrist to signal an image Ruth could visualize. Almost as a reflex action she visualized the pain medication dripping into her intravenous line.

Ruth was very responsive to Gary's touch, but she also did well spontaneously, on her own. She would visualize herself in a Jacuzzi, with all the bubbles and the hot water milling around her and the pain going away. Or she would visualize being at the beach, looking up at the clouds and the different cumulus cloud formations, fusing them into various shapes and objects like balloons to elevate her immune system. Visualizing things like the Jacuzzi and the summer sun on the beach brought heat to her legs. Her leg temperature was down to about 80 degrees because of faulty circulation, but when she visualized the sun, and sunbathing, all oiled up, hot and sweaty, the temperature in her legs would shoot up to 98 degrees. It got so she would just think of the color red and become warm. The psychologist, Dr. Archer, would hook up the biofeedback to Ruth's feet and toes, and with a thermistor to register her body temperature, together they would visualize to increase the blood flow to her extremities.

For her arthritis, Ruth would visualize an erupting volcano, its lava washing away all the toxins in her body. She also envisioned artists painting over bright red walls—her inflamed intestines—with white paint to cool them off. Her intestines got very irritated from some of the medications she took, and using white over the bright red got rid of the irritation. White is also a healing color. Ruth was rated in the top 10 percent of the population for suggestibility, and this boded well for her continued improvement. Under hypnotic suggestion she once detached from her body pain for 24 hours.

With all that had been done, there were still few significant changes inside Ruth, but she never gave up. She was a fighter.

Her face had always looked well, even when her body didn't, but we were bringing the two together with exercise and massage. And nothing was wrong with her mind—she thought clearly. Supported by their church, Ruth and Gary also brought a new understanding to many of the people in the church about how to deal with chronic illness and not lose your patience or your faith. Ruth is well into the process of getting well from a situation nobody normally gets well from. *Someone must have listened.*

I looked at Ruth. She looked years younger than her age, her face was radiant, her eyes sparkling at the promise of a new and useful life. Gary looked at her with pride. And I knew my parents and my Aunt Belle would be proud of her and the church that gave her their unstinting love and support.

A Search for Meaning

If I take the wings of the morning,
And dwell in the uttermost parts
of the sea,
Even there thy hand shall lead me,
And thy right hand shall hold me.

—PSALM 139:9-10

He was good-looking, young, single and successful. And he couldn't believe what the doctor was saying.

"I've only got two years to live?"

"At the most. Six months to two years."

The neurologist had done a few tests, including an MRI, and concluded Jeff Rich had a brain tumor. As Jeff sat there, stunned, the doctor mentioned in an impersonal way the

121

stages he would be going through. Jeff had no reason to doubt him. The man was a highly qualified neurologist.

"I wasn't going to get off easily," Jeff later told me. "First, I would lose control of my right side coordination. Next, my sight would begin to fail. I would be able to see but I wouldn't be able to tell what I was seeing. This would happen within the first few days. There was more, but I was too numb to take it all in. I finally said, thinking there must be a ray of hope somewhere, 'Is there anything good at all?'

"'No,' the doctor said, 'there's nothing good I can see.' He stood up and opened the door, and out I went. 'Good luck,' he said.

"Good luck. It was the most unbelievable few moments of my life. Only a week before I had been telling myself how lucky I was. A few days later I was having some numbness in my right arm and hand. Then I got a pulsing that ran down my spine and my left arm. It would come and go. I didn't think too much about it. Later I was driving down the street and this trembling came over me: the shakes, only worse. I controlled the car with an effort. I knew something was wrong and I was frightened. For the first time in my adult life something was happening to me that I had no control over. It was devastating."

After the visit to the doctor, Jeff wandered around for hours, telling himself it hadn't happened. He was too young, too vital. This kind of thing happened to other people, older people, not people like him. Like him? Like what? That was a thought. He wasn't sure who he was. He was 33, and he'd made a lot of money in business, and had a lot of fun knocking around the world, dating beautiful women, enjoying himself. If this was the end, no one would be able to write a good obituary about him. He hadn't done anything to be remembered by.

A couple of days later he got a bill from the neurologist and wondered if the doctor was trying to tell him something. He hadn't wasted any time.

I knew Jeff almost as well as I knew my own sons. I had taken an interest in him from childhood. I was both his friend and his doctor. He called me the next day at home and left his name and number.

I was away for the weekend. When I returned, I called him back and learned what had happened. I was concerned and called for copies of the tests he had taken. By the time I called Jeff back, I had read enough to allow me at least to be reassuring. I could be wrong, but he knew me well enough to know I was not given to platitudes.

"Jeff," I said, "don't get too uptight. I had a dream about you and I know you're going to be okay. In that dream, I was helping a child to find his way home. I was leading him by the hand."

That child was Jeff. With four sons of my own, I had symbolized him as a son too. He was very dear to me.

Jeff didn't know what to say. It would have been laughable under any other circumstance, except he had known and looked up to me all his life. He knew I wasn't playing games with him. He had never done anything that I hadn't been supportive of, and at this point, I was his only support. We decided he should have another opinion. He made an appointment with a neurosurgeon, but the diagnosis of a tumor was the same and surgery was scheduled. Jeff later described it:

"They cut into my skull to relieve the pressure on the brain, but they didn't get into the brain. After surgery, an oncologist suggested radiation and chemotherapy. I talked to Gladys and we decided I wasn't going to have any of that, not right then."

Jeff may have had a premonition. "Before any of this happened I had decided that if I ever got cancer, I would not do chemo or radiation. I'd seen people get cancer, and some of them didn't get well with chemo and radiation. Some do get well, others don't, that's a fact. Even if they choose chemo and radiation, they should combine it with alternative therapies and contact the physician within for the best chance for wellness. Instead, treatment tore down their bodies, and all the fight seemed to go out of them."

Jeff came back to me and I reminded him of the physician within. He was willing to do anything feasible if his inner voice told him it was right. He started meditating and visualizing. He felt that the oncologist and the radiation therapist were limiting his options. Their primary suggestion in the way of therapy was radiation, but he had this dream that said just the opposite. He dreamt he was outside a room that was kind of boxed in. He could see out through a one-way mirror, but other people couldn't see in. He saw somebody, a man or a woman, sitting in front of some instrument. All of a sudden two dogs bounded in and viciously attacked this person. The dogs left and the person got up and walked past where Jeff was sitting. He couldn't tell if the person had been injured or not, not unless this person's clothes were removed so Jeff could see what was underneath. He saw this as a message. Some doctors claimed that the radiation techniques were so specific they could knock out the tumor without damaging any other tissue. The dream was saying that unless we got below the surface, we wouldn't know if healthy tissue had been damaged or not. Jeff opted not to have the radiation. I couldn't, in good conscience, tell him what to do. Jeff made his own decision. The physician within was speaking.

Why else had he had the dream? He wasn't ready to die. He had just come off a hard relationship with a young woman he cared about. He had been depressed. He had taken stock of his life, and decided there had to be more to living than having fun and making money. Something was lacking and he talked it over with me. When he mentioned meditating, developing spiritually, I was encouraging. When he wanted to change to a macrobiotic diet, I got a book on macrobiotic cooking and gave it to him.

He took to watching people. They all appeared to be getting on with their lives: marrying, changing jobs, going to parties, planning trips. Here he was on some strange diet, eating alone, not enjoying his food, his weight dropping from a slim 165 pounds to an emaciated 135 pounds. His clothes hung on him like a hall tree, his cheeks were pale and gaunt, and his elbows and knees were as sharp as knives. He had been so good-looking he was accustomed to young women looking at him on the street and in restaurants. But nobody was looking now except older people with a sympathetic eye.

He retreated into a world all his own.

"I was totally focused on staying alive. I kept thinking of Gladys's dream. She had always been right with me medically and I had a feeling she was intuitive. She was right about so many things other people were confused about. I tried to meditate and remain calm, as she suggested, and keep my mind off the tumor in my head. 'Don't think about it,' Gladys said. 'Don't give it any food for thought.'"

That made sense to Jeff. He started to travel, no great distances, to macrobiotic conferences—until he tired of brown rice. He meditated at a Buddhist monastery near San Francisco. "I tried so hard to stay calm it made me nervous. I was off sugar and I didn't drink. I went off meat, too, and ate some rice and vegetables. When I dropped down to the lightweight class I went back to Gladys and told her I didn't think I was eating right."

I had been waiting for him to come back after going his way. I had confidence in his resilience. I put him on the Cayce diet for gaining strength and weight. "You've done a great job cleaning out your system. Now is the time to build your strength." I charted a diet for him: fish and fowl, green vegetables like Swiss chard, broccoli, green beans, heavy lettuce, fresh fruits, and the basic vitamins—B-complex, A, C, E and D, with sunshine and fresh air.

He realized he hadn't been doing anything truly important with his life and he talked about that. "I had made a lot of money, but what good was it when you had one foot in the cemetery and another in a quagmire? I was beginning to think that that was my real trouble, and what, ironically, my rational brain was telling me. And it had acted up to make sure I listened. I needed to take time to know why I was on this planet. I needed a purpose, something to justify my existence. I needed to help others and to create something useful—even if that something was a sustaining love with another human being, an unselfish and caring love for the sake of love. For the first time I felt my life coming together. I stopped thinking about the tumor. The physician within that Gladys spoke of was beginning to stir about in my head.

"I began to think of wellness, not sickness. I took greater notice of people in my meditations, getting a new understanding of how they were living and why they were dying. In my wanderings I watched people die. It was not easy. I saw a nun who had breast cancer die with a smile. She was at peace, convinced she was going to another and better world. I made friends with a younger woman at a macrobiotic conference. I soon saw she had no tight hold on life. She had nothing to live for, and so nothing to go on for. It didn't mean that everyone dies who has nothing to live for, but it does make it a lot easier."

A doctor friend of mine asked Jeff: "Do you live alone?" Jeff said yes.

"I didn't even have a dog. I felt an emptiness. You've got to have someone, even a dog. I found you have to love something to keep going. I learned the hard way. Is there another way?"

The door was open. He spoke to me about goals. "Yes," I said, "we all need something to dream about and wake up to each morning."

Jeff had a feeling of elation. He was digging into himself, finding he wasn't all that bad off. He wasn't in pain. He had stopped thinking of the tumor. Occasionally, when the thought did seep in, he saw the tumor as a benign friend telling him he had to turn his life around. He gave thanks for his continuing health and wholeness.

Jeff discovered the wisdom of leaving things after they served a purpose—like the macrobiotic diet. It may have seemed a small thing to some, but it came as a great awakening to him. His brain with all its problems was subject to his will. It was as if the brain were saying, "I didn't get this tumor to scare you. You get something out of everything you pay a price for."

He could hear the words forming in his brain. They were so clear. One day he looked in the mirror and said, "You don't have to do this diet anymore. Live in the world, not away from it, dine with your friends, get back to living a normal life. Forget the tumor, except to bless it for waking you. Look on it as a friend. Take care of your life. You've relieved yourself of a life-time of bad karma in seven months of cleansing and replenishing your body and mind. Now move on. Think of yourself as well. As you leave it, so too will the tumor leave you. It will have no place in your body."

Jeff resumed his life, eating whatever he wanted, green salads, fresh fruits, occasionally fish or poultry. He didn't make anything out of his diet. It was casual, he was casual. He took long walks, breathing deeply of the great outdoors, the mountain and desert air. Every breath infused him with new life and energy.

He communicated with his tumor in his visualizations. "I would close my eyes and relax. I'd see the tumor breaking up in little cells and moving out of my skull. I put a white light around it. White light is healing. I wanted the tumor to heal itself as it was moving out. I saw it in my mind's eye, breaking apart, like bubbles on the surface of a pool."

Jeff meditated every day for a year at my suggestion. It got so he enjoyed it. He saw it was working. The tumor was no longer a villainous stranger threatening his life. It had been transformed by his visualizations into a benevolent visitor who would do as he was told to do.

As Jeff improved he reduced the meditations to once or twice a week. He checked in with the neurosurgeon every three to six months. He thought so seldom of his illness that he sometimes forgot to make his appointments. When the neurosurgeon does MRIs of his brain, Jeff is philosophical about it.

"They go in and take a picture. They see the brain from nearly every aspect, and they see the tumor. But it doesn't do anything anymore. It just never had done anything again. First you see a spot, a dark spot. Then you realize it's really a light spot with a dark background. It's not malignant. They say it can become malignant at any time, but it hasn't and it won't. I am confident of that. I'm very calm as I look at the picture. I think of Christ, who has been so close to me as I've lived with this experience, an experience designed to test my reason for being and make me realize how precious each moment is. I needed to get hold of my life and make it mean something."

I had heard words like this before in inspirational talks and seen a speaker's eyes light up. But I had never seen a glow like I now saw on Jeff's face.

"This tumor," he said, "was an answer to a prayer."

An answer to a prayer? I looked at him. I thought for a moment he had been dwelling altogether too much on everything he had gone through.

He saw my look and laughed. "No, I'm not off my rocker. We haven't talked about faith and prayer, or my strong belief in Christ. I'm not a great churchgoer. I don't spend my days talking to Jesus. But three months before I got sick, sitting home alone, I had an overpowering impulse to pray to Jesus. My life had been drifting and I didn't have much enthusiasm for the way I was living it. So I decided I'd have a little impromptu chat with Jesus.

"I spoke to Jesus like I was talking to a friend. I was sure he wouldn't mind. He hadn't been a stickler for formality or ceremony, walking around as he did in sandals and a simple robe in all kinds of weather. 'Dear Jesus,' I said, 'if you are to be real in my life, let me know. Whatever it is, it'll be okay. Just let me know. I can handle it.'"

Jeff's face had become radiant as he went back to that day. "As I look back I realize something must have been stirring inside me, some premonition. I went on and said, 'This is a nice life I have, and I know it. I have the best of everything that money can buy. But if you can't show me what I'm doing here, take me home, because it all seems like a big waste of time. I don't know what I'm doing. I don't know why I'm here. I don't know where to go with this life of mine. Please tell me.'"

And what did Jesus say?

Jeff smiled. "He said a lot. I remember thinking of it, as I sat shaking in that neurologist's office while he told me, without any feeling, about all these bad things that were going to happen. I remember thinking to myself, 'Ah, now I know God's intention. The tumor was no accident. It was all meant to be. And put me on a path that will give me the answers to my questions.'

"I truly believed God was working in his wondrous way. Talking to Jesus was like talking to God. I had a strong connection with God and Christ. In my late teens, I was encouraged to build my relationship with God and to be of service. 'That's why we're here,' I was told. But over the years, with socializing, working at my job and doing well, some of that connection slipped out of my life. Now it was flooding back into my consciousness, making me more aware than ever about doing for others. I found myself thanking God for this tumor that made me stop and think long enough to turn my life around. It's like I'd lived on the razor edge of life, then had edged over into a promised land where there were no bounds or limitations. I had something to say now that I never really had to say before. When I talked to somebody before, I never felt that I came from a position of any knowledge. Now it was like I had a new insight. Like I knew what it was to have lived, died, then come back. It was as if I had almost died a hundred times, and yet still lived, with all the light that comes from a close brush with death, reliving in a moment everything that had ever happened to me. From this life that had no purpose spilled out every misdeed, every mistake."

He tapped his head ever so lightly. "And now I've got my head on straight. Finally."

This search for meaning was something I had observed elsewhere in humanity adrift, and I knew it meant different things to different people. Jeff was thinking now of extending himself, getting back into higher education, preparing for what he wanted to do: large-scale communications that would break down barriers. The tumor had served its purpose. He could go wherever his brain and heart would take him.

"I need fulfillment," he told me, "and to do something useful in a world in crisis. I need to help people of all creeds to communicate with one another."

I nodded. "To know where you're going you have to know where you're at. So now that you know where you're at, you can't go back."

He knew what I meant.

"Yes," he said. "I've fought to be where I am. I won't soon forget how I got there."

The Secret of Survival

Surely the weak shall perish,
And only the fit survive.

—ROBERT SERVICE

There's hardly a day I don't learn something from a patient. Sometimes it's patience: An elderly man calmly waits for an organ transplant with one eye on the calendar. Sometimes it's courage: A child hobbles about on one leg, smiling and laughing; or a young mother slugs it out with cancer, so she can have still another day with the child who needs her.

Then there was Donna Franquemont, a nurse and my patient for 15 years, giving of herself to the husband she loved, nursing his last years as though the honeymoon had never

131

ended. She was always cheerful and calm, her life illuminated by a mind-boggling exposure to the boundless power of the human spirit. She was doing graduate work in nutrition at the University of Iowa when the war abruptly ended in the summer of 1945 and the hospital quickly emptied itself of the sick and disabled. She was overwhelmed. It was something she would never forget.

"After four long years of fear, personal hardship and rationing (especially of young men), the hospital patients and personnel erupted into one colossal binge. You would walk into a ward in which 20 patients were jammed the day before, and no one was there. Everyone was in the hallways, coming and going, jumping up and down. When you saw someone you knew—doctor, nurse, dietitian or patient—you hugged them, screamed and became ecstatic.

"The hospital doors were thrown open and everyone came or left as they pleased. Needless to say, alcohol flowed like water. It seemed like everyone was imbibing but those of us engaged in research. We didn't want to do anything to disturb the alcohol content of our blood samples—which we were working with in the lab."

It was a day to remember. Then something else happened that was engraved on Donna's brain and helped shape the rest of a long and fruitful life. It gave her an insight that may have made her days considerably longer and productive.

She could hardly believe her eyes as she saw the patients on the hospital's critical list the night before now roll out of their beds and head for home. Some of them hadn't been given another 24 hours to live.

"They were whistling and cheering. They didn't even check with their doctors or nurses. They just jumped to their feet, threw on some clothes, and sailed out into the street, with huge grins on their faces, looking for any vehicle that would get them home."

Out of curiosity Donna stopped one of the patients at the hospital door, a middle-aged woman. Donna saw a light in her eyes, the sparkle of youth. She was radiant, moving as though she was in an altered state of consciousness. The years of care had dropped away.

"Last night you were at death's door," Donna said to her. "And now you're well and on your way home. What happened?"

The woman edged closer to the door. "You're too young to understand. The war's over. Life's beginning. My boys will be home. After four years of being stifled and afraid I've got something to live for."

Something to live for. It rang a bell. It was a lesson that Donna retained all these years, into her 70s. She always set a goal for herself, something to shoot for, something to keep her interested in the next day and the day after, on into the ever dwindling future. Her enthusiasm and her concern for those less fortunate than herself kept her going. She stayed useful, never leaning on anyone and always keeping alive the physician within that made her healthy and optimistic, sure of herself and who she was. Never hemmed in by the shibboleths of the past, Donna lived for the present and the future. There would always be a future for people who believed as she did, and there were many like her: the survivors.

I had often groped about for the secret of survival myself. I thought I had found it in the elderly ladies who had gathered around the mystic Edgar Cayce in Virginia Beach, the ones who used his castor oil packs for their rheumy muscles, and a lotion of peanut oil, olive oil and lanolin that kept their octogenarian faces wrinkle-free. They were tough and gentle. So too was Olive Landers, the ageless sweet-faced woman dashing about to gather notes for her column in the Cayce newsletter. Struck down by an errant driver one night while crossing the street, she was dragged 200 yards along the pavement. She was 90 at the time. Many of her bones were broken, and her internal injuries were multiple. I was sure I would never see her again. Yet three or four months later, on a visit to Virginia Beach, I saw this tiny figure hurtling toward me with a pad and pencil in hand. It was Olive Landers. She was all business. Before I could comment on her recovery, she said with a bright smile, "Do you have any news for me? It's been a slow week."

She was the greatest news of the day, and she didn't even know it—typical of survivors. The last person they thought about was themselves.

I saw so many survivors and often helped them stay that way. They were like a Detroit assembly line—almost endless. Occasionally, I'd get one who toughed it out on his or her own.

A new patient that I hadn't seen before came into my office, sat down and announced she was 83 years old. Then she said, "I don't like doctors. I don't go to doctors. I haven't seen a doctor in 67 years."

I gave her a second look, and I believed her. There wasn't any "give" in Betty Jane. She had a seamed face, like the old pioneers, her lips pinched together. "I've never gone to anyone for help before."

I said okay. What else was there to say? Her voice had a rattle in it, and I suspected there was something wrong with her lungs. I didn't have to bring out my stethoscope to know the woman had a serious chest congestion. A closer examination with the stethoscope showed she had pneumonia. While I was checking her chest I noticed she had a large mass in her right breast. The moment the stethoscope touched her chest, she said, "I know that's cancer and you're not going to take it out."

"How long have you had that thing?"

She said, "Ten years."

"Wow, 10 years. How have you kept it under control like this?"

Betty Jane shrugged. "Every time it starts to grow, I say, 'Stop it,' and it stops."

We looked at each other, taking stock.

"That's great," I said. "Why don't you think it away?"

She hadn't thought about that, so I talked to her about visualizing, and focusing the visualization on her breast to help the cancer go away. I thought I'd have to work on her a bit, but she surprised me—she was a real survivor and she decided it was a great idea—as long as she was visualizing her own way. She liked the idea of a physician within her taking hold of things. It meant she didn't need an outsider, some doctor who would be curing her. She'd be getting rid of that nasty old cancer herself, and that made it all right.

I didn't see Betty Jane for another six months. When she came back, the cancer mass was about half the size it had been. I saw her in another six months and it was down somewhat more. I could see she had been working on it, but she didn't want to talk about it. It was something she was doing herself and wasn't properly my concern. After all, she was the lady who hadn't seen a doctor in 67 years. I wasn't about to argue the point, not while she was so spunky and improving.

I didn't see her for two years. When she came in for a checkup, I took one look at her and said, "Betty Jane, what are you doing with this thing? It's still the same size. It hasn't changed a millimeter since you were last here."

By now she was 87 years old. She just shrugged her shoulders and said, "Oh, I got tired of fussing with it. I gave it one last visualization to stay as it was, then I forgot about it. That thing will never kill me."

I believed her. She spoke with such conviction and that was half the battle—it was mind over mass. Cancer would never kill her. Perhaps she'd fall down a bunch of stairs and die, but that mess on her chest would never do it. That's how she thought about it—the mess, and not a mass.

Five years passed. I often thought of this old martinet, but I never worried about her. Betty Jane wasn't the kind you worried about. One day, she strolled into my office without making an appointment. She was 92 now, yet she looked the same as when we had first met: the furrowed face, the iron-gray hair swept back tight to her head, the thin pale strip of a mouth, the square jaw.

She was still going strong. She had no more problems with her lungs, and the cancer was just about the same size as it had been the last time. "I'm not fussing with my breast at all," she told me. "It's not that important." I had an idea that she had just come in to let me know how well she was doing, and that she didn't need a doctor after all. I was right.

A week or two later I got a little note from Betty Jane. "Thanks for what you've done. And for putting that physician inside me to work." It was quite an acknowledgment, coming from someone like Betty Jane.

Six or seven years have passed since then. Any day now, I'm sure, she'll come walking in—probably on her 100th birthday— just so she can say, "Pay that old mess no mind, Dr. Gladys. It's sticking around to keep me company."

I'm fond of talking about these people because they're something of an inspiration to me and everyone who knows them. I also have a number of inspiring elderly patients, in their 80s and 90s, who are mentally very alert. None have Alzheimer's or senile dementia. All have a great zest for living. Two of my patients got to talking in my waiting room. One woman was 96 and the other woman was 88. The 88-year-old said something to the 96-year-old about their being the same age. And the 96-year-old said, "Oh, I think I'm older than you are." The 88-year-old was absolutely amazed. "But you look so young," she said. And they had a good laugh.

In the past year, the same 96-year-old had had two surgical procedures, but they didn't slow her down. She put a course together for the Scottsdale Presbyterian Church dealing with words from the Bible, and did a discussion on these words and concepts in such a way that her class became very popular. When she finished it, the minister asked if he could put this information together in a form that could be used in other provinces of the Presbyterian church. Though she has trouble getting around and has a number of physical problems, her desire to be of help and to continue to teach has not diminished with the years.

Another patient of mine, who is 92, has been coming in for 30 years. Through the years she has worried about the wrinkles on her face, but has kept right on living her life to the fullest. She has always walked a lot. Until recently, she was walking between two and five miles a day. About 10 years ago a car ran over her. She came into my office with bruises starting at her right ankle and going right on up to her left shoulder. The muscles and tissues were badly bruised but there were no broken bones. She recovered from this accident fairly well. Two years later she developed a cancer in the left breast and had to have a mastectomy. Every time she comes into my office she's got something interesting to tell me. Last spring she came in and said that she was one of the finalists in a Readers Digest sweepstakes and she was certain that she was going to win. Her question for me was: If she got to go on TV, would I mind if she talked about the work that we were doing. I laughed and told her to go ahead. I'd go on the show with her.

I also have as patients a couple in their mid-80s. They had 10 children and I don't know how many grandchildren and great-grandchildren. They had a family reunion where there were 50 people, and that didn't count all their great-grandchildren. The wife told me that her husband's mother, widowed, had eloped when she was 82 and lived another 10 years, happily married to the man she eloped with. When somebody asked why she had eloped, she sniffed and said, "I didn't want a big fuss."

Only recently a couple in their 80s came in for a physical. They were leaving to head up a tour group which was going to Alaska. The tour was to last three weeks. They have led tours for many years and were continuing to do so despite physical problems and things which would hold other people back. They did all of the scheduling for the tour, all the booking, all the arrangements for cabins and flights. They took full responsibility.

Another lady in her mid-80s was one of the people going on the tour with this couple. She came into my office about three years ago, incapacitated with abdominal pain after many surgeries, and suffering from severe intestinal obstruction. We used castor oil packs, dietary changes and massage until she got to feeling much better and went on to take the tour. When I first saw her I sent her for a massage with John Marshall. When he started massaging her, she began sobbing. He came running across the hall and asked me to come over, thinking that maybe he had done something to hurt her. I went across the hall and discovered what was bothering her. Five people in her family had died in the last year and a half, and she had been unable to cry. When the masseur began working with her, it was as if he touched some place inside of her that opened the floodgates of grief. She was crying now for the first time and releasing this pent-up emotion. Since that time she has gotten progressively more healthy. She has a home on about an acre of land that has all kinds of fruit trees on it, and aside from some help from a grandson, she pretty much takes care of her own work.

She reminded me of my Aunt Belle, one of my great inspirations. In the early '70s, the time of the hippie generation, a lot of American young people were going over to India to find a "guru."

The Indian government really was not at all happy about this influx of young American people who came to India, ran out of money, and ended up like the many people in India who were already having trouble finding enough food and clothing to keep themselves going.

There were two young men who came to the children's home where Aunt Belle was taking care of the children of leper parents. Aunt Belle took in these two men because she felt sorry for them and she thought maybe they could help her a little bit with the children she was caring for. The people in the city of Dehra Dun were unhappy about these young people being there and they sent the police out to check on them one night. Aunt Belle had already gone to bed when the police came to the door and asked these two young Americans for their passports. One of them readily handed his over but the other one, for some obscure reason, refused to do so. This infuriated the police, so they not only took those boys into custody, but proceeded to take all the children in the home off to a Hindu school. There were about 95 children in the home at the time, and every one of them was removed. Aunt Belle was still asleep upstairs and knew nothing of what was going on. Some of the children ran out the back and escaped into the jungle, but the rest of them were taken to the school.

When Aunt Belle came downstairs in the morning, she found no one there. The place was empty and she couldn't imagine what had happened. After a while the children who had escaped into the jungle behind the home came straggling in one at a time and told her what had taken place. She was devastated and really didn't know what to do. She prayed about it, and over a period of three months most of the children came back and she was able to go on with her work.

My brother Carl came to visit her six months after this incident. When he was ready to leave she walked to the door with him. She stopped, looked at herself, and said to Carl, "Oh my, look at me. I'm all bent over." She continued, "God has helped me through worse times than this. He'll certainly help me through this one." With a mighty crunching of bones she straightened her body up and grew about two inches as she claimed her place in God's kingdom and his continuing work. She was 90 at the time.

It is pleasant to think of people getting better as they get older, especially when one is getting older oneself. I thought of this as I sat across the desk from an elderly woman with a serene and alert expression. She had lost several members of her family within a brief period, and I remembered her as the woman who had cried so profoundly while being massaged. I reminded her of the incident.

"Yes," she said, without flinching. "I lost them all. They all died at once. Two sisters, a brother, a son, and my daughter-in-law."

I looked for signs of depression but saw none. She was widowed and 85, but she looked years younger. You could see the indomitable will in her eyes. She came from a medical family—her husband and a brother had both been surgeons. Her name was Nadine Patterson. She had been a registered nurse for years, heading the nursing staff at a Phoenix hospital. She had survived cancer surgery with the help of her husband. Remembering this, she smiled. "He wouldn't let the doctors give me anything, not even a blood transfusion. He said, 'Let her replenish her own blood.' And I did."

Nadine took care of her mother and father when they were dying. Of her two sisters, one died of cancer, the other of a heart attack. They were in the hospital at the same time. "Then," Nadine went on to say, "two weeks after I buried one sister, my only son was in an automobile accident and was killed. His wife died the next year. I took in their son, my grandson, who I've raised since then. He's 26 years old now."

I looked at the weathered face, the head held erect with pride. How had she done it all?

"I have great faith. I get up in the morning and the first thing I do is walk out on my patio and say, 'Thank you, God, for another day. Thank you for letting me live one more day in this world.' He helped me through all of it. You've got to ask. If you ask, he will deliver."

I smiled. "I'm afraid he'd get bored with me."

"Well, he probably gets bored with me. I just happen to have a disposition that holds on. It's been that way all my life. I've always had something I had to do for someone, always had someone to care for. When I was nine years old, my mother was very ill. She had a nervous breakdown after my father died. My mother was with her sister in Phoenix, and I was back in Oklahoma where we came from. So it was up to me to take my brothers and sisters on the train from Oklahoma City to Arizona. There were five of us. I carried the little one that was two, and I had the one that was six years old hold on to the one that was three. And we managed the other one between us. That's the way we traveled until we got off the train. I remember the conductor asking, 'Who's in charge of all these kids?' And I answered, 'I'm in charge.'"

She's been in charge ever since. A registered nurse since she was 20, Nadine graduated from high school when she was 16, worked for the government taking care of the poor and super-vised surgery at a Phoenix hospital. Her husband, Dr. John Harris Patterson, had been dead for 30 years when I first met her. He had been a conventional surgeon, but he was also homeopathic and holistic in his inclination. "He was a gall bladder specialist," Nadine told me. "After he did a gall bladder operation, he would ask his patients to take a teaspoon of white Karo syrup with a little orange juice every morning for the rest of their lives. 'Take this,' he said, 'and you'll never have a liver problem.'"

Nadine took everything one day at a time, and her philosophy was: "Nobody ever promised me a rose garden." The day we spoke, she had driven over to the clinic by herself because there was simply no one to drive her. She had recently been on an ocean cruise and when she returned, she decided to have an eye test. The doctor thought she might be developing glaucoma and he gave her some eye drops, but she was allergic to them. "I got violently ill," Nadine told me. "I lost 30 pounds and had a bloated stomach that ached something awful. A friend in California who wrote a lot about allergies told me, 'If you're allergic to it, it'll kill you. Get off it.'"

She could barely walk, but she made it in to see me.

"I knew how sick I was," she later said, "but I didn't know what it was. The wonderful thing was that Dr. Gladys didn't concentrate on the sickness, but on me, even when I said to her, 'I think I'm two steps from the mortuary.' Dr. Gladys just laughed and said, 'Come on, let's get you started back on the road.'"

I gave Nadine a shot of vitamin B-complex and then had John Marshall give her a therapeutic massage. Then I prescribed castor oil packs for her abdomen. "Believe it or not," Nadine later recalled, "after two of them my belly stopped aching and went down to its normal size. Dr. Gladys also had me x-rayed. When I was being x-rayed, the technician said, 'You've had so many operations, I can't get a clear picture.' I'd had 15 operations, one thing after another. There simply wasn't that much inside me to x-ray.

"Now I'm walking around and driving, without pain. There was a time I was so bloated with gas that I couldn't even scream.

"Dr. Gladys gives you confidence. You really get to thinking that you do have a physician within, as well as outside, you."

Only once did this patient falter—that day on the massage table. Being only too human, her physician within finally released the tension building up inside her from the grief that had contributed to her illness. But even then her faith was not shaken. Nadine remembered: "I got down on my knees and said, 'Why, Lord, did you have to take them all at once and leave me here all alone?'"

And what was the answer? *Was* there an answer? "There's always an answer," Nadine replied. "God does not give you any more than you can carry. He poured it on me pretty badly, but he knew I could handle it. You can get depressed and say, 'Woe is me,' and feel sorry for yourself. Or you can get in there and fight. I saw it all as a challenge, and I blessed God for it. I have had a wonderful life. And it's just beginning in some ways. Since I found the physician within."

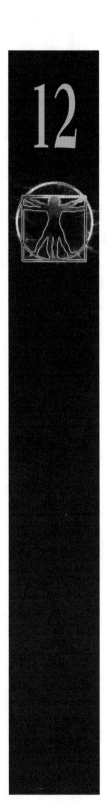

Follow Your Dreams

I often have this strange and moving dream of an unknown woman
Who I love, and who loves me.

—Paul Verlaine

Dreams are a link to reality. With dreams, the subconscious mind makes contact with the conscious mind. We dream every night, whether we remember it or not. People deprived of sleep have a problem because they have lost dreaming time. Dreams are good for the human psyche, keeping it in balance and sometimes releasing what some call an inner "dis-ease" or psychosis.

Most people don't pay any attention to their dreams and soon forget them. But if we didn't dream, we'd be in trouble. Dreams are our connections between our inner and outer worlds, and they are often our guides.

I believe that nothing happens to us in our conscious life that has not been previewed in our dreams. Thomas Edison visualized the phonograph and the motion picture projector while nodding off. Robert Louis Stevenson saw the unfolding story of *Treasure Island* in a dream.

We would be better guided in life if we not only remembered our dreams, but learned how to interpret them. It doesn't require a genius. The symbolism is simple and best explained by the dreamer whose mind created them. They are often prophetic—like Jeff Rich's dream after his brain tumor appeared, and my own dream that he would be all right. And only a few days before his assassination, Abraham Lincoln dreamed that he saw his body lying in state in the White House. When he told his cabinet about it, they all demurred. He was the only one who believed it.

Everyone and everything in a dream are parts of the dreamer. Every person in your dream is a manifestation of some aspect of yourself. Every fixture in the dream speaks of something going on in your subconscious. Tables, chairs, windows, oceans, sky, hair, eyes, ears, limbs—all of these are part of what your unconscious mind is trying to bring forward to consciousness. All symbols have a special meaning for you. By concentrating you can figure out what they signify.

A person we dream about represents some characteristic within ourselves that we're trying to deal with. In our dreams, we are the producers, the actors, the stagehands and the props. Every part of the dream scenario has something to do with what's going on inside us at an unconscious level. And there are many different kinds of dreams: precognitive dreams, health dreams, guidance dreams, healing dreams—both for physical and emotional disturbances.

A dream may seem silly, like a pink cow on a purple moon, or appear totally irrelevant to what we're concerned with in our conscious lives. But if we write down our dreams, we will both remember more of our dreams, and understand better their symbolism. Even when we don't think we remember dreams, they often play out in our conscious life.

Some of life's events are as symbolic and meaningful as any dream could be. As a physician, a dream often gives me insight into what I can expect, particularly in the delivery of a baby. I encourage my obstetric patients to put their dreams on paper before they get up in the morning or talk about them. Even the nurses working with me have taken to dreaming about birthing situations.

During her pregnancy, a nurse in her 20s remained very active, working at our clinic until her seventh month, when she developed severe asthma. I told her to stop working and rest, but she insisted on staying on the job. She began to concentrate on invoking her dreams. She meditated each night before she went to bed, and she placed a pad with a pencil on her night table. This way she encouraged the visualization and subconscious dream process. The first night she began doing this was a horror. Soon after her eyes closed, a dream started. She saw her baby in a casket, wrapped in a plastic bag. She put her hands over her eyes in the dream and walked away, but, as though hypnotized, she found herself compelled to return to the casket.

As she looked down at the child his eyes opened, and he said, "Do I know you?"

She grasped the dream child's meaning. She had been so busy with her work and whatever activities she had, she hadn't found time to connect with the baby she was bringing into the world. The dream was more effective than anything I could say or do. She stopped working in the clinic that day. Two months later she delivered a healthy, normal baby. A boy. Which she had foreseen.

I have found over the years that the way to get guidance in a dream is to make the best conscious decision I can regarding a particular question for which I am seeking an answer. I'll say, "Okay, God, this is what I've decided. Is it right?" Then I wait and see what answer I get in the way of a dream. If the dream is straight ahead—green lights, green pastures, sunny skies—then I go ahead with the decision I made. If, on the other hand, the dream depicts a total disaster—a car wreck, a building on fire, floodgates opening up—I will back up, change my decision and say, "Okay, is this better?" Then I wait and see what I get in the way of still another dream. There have been times when, in spite of getting an answer that could be interpreted negatively, I've gone ahead with my decision and usually I've been sorry that I did.

You get to know yourself better with visualization, dreams and exercise. We don't give our bodies credit enough for being able to communicate what is going on in our deeper being. Especially sensitive when it is under duress, the body cries out for the help the conscious mind has denied it.

One patient of mine, a young woman with a history of severe headaches, was an expert at denial. We did everything we could for her: biofeedback, manipulations, massage, exercises. Then we talked about diet. At this she turned her head away. She wasn't interested. That should have been a clue, but we weren't that alert to her signals. She herself, at her wit's end, finally resolved the problem—subconsciously. Trying to contact the physician in a dream state, she had a dream that hit so directly on her problem that a child could have interpreted it. She was sitting in my examining room when she told me about it. She had a sheepish look on her face, and another of her headaches.

"Dr. Gladys," she said, "will you listen to a dream?"

"Gladly," I said, having no idea what was coming.

"In this dream," she said, pursing her lips, looking a little uncomfortable, "I was sitting in your examining room—this room—suffering from one of my headaches. I reached into my bag for some pills."

She put them in the palm of her hand and was about to take them when in the dream I walked into the examining room and barked in an authoritative voice, "Don't take them."

She had two pieces of chocolate in her hands, two M&Ms. She had been snitching chocolate. I didn't know about it, and neither did anyone else in the clinic. In her dream she looked at me like an errant child caught with her hand in the cookie jar. And she pleaded *mea culpa*.

We now knew where the headaches were coming from. She was allergic to chocolate. We had never tested her for that, and she had kept it to herself. The physician within told her chocolate was the cause and she shied away from mentioning it. But she couldn't keep it hidden from her subconscious mind, or from the physician within, represented by me in her dream. We all knew now what she subconsciously knew. It was up to her to stop eating chocolate. I couldn't order her, but she knew what my feelings were. She was a grown person. She could no longer complain about a headache and get any sympathy.

We're never too young or too old to dream, or to benefit from dreams. Some of our dreams track back through a lifetime, explaining a disease or disability which might otherwise go unexplained.

Significant dreams come to those who are ready for them. Carol Osman Brown, journalist and winner of more than 50 awards, including the Sweepstakes Award from the National Federation of Press Women, started dreaming after I gave her a dream log. "Until then," she says, "I had a hard time interpreting the dreams and getting insight into my life. After a while, with tips from Gladys, my physician for 30 years, I got the hang of it. The recurring dreams were the most impactive on my life. In this one dream I saw a large tree. In its many branches there were lots of children giggling and dancing. I saw the sun filtering through the trees. It gave a golden glow to the children waving for me to climb the tree. They appeared to be waiting for me, with warm smiles on their friendly faces. I had an idea this was telling me I should be writing children's books, in addition to the journalistic work that brought me some recognition. I discussed it with Gladys and she agreed with my interpretation. I applied myself to the books for children and was not only successful, but found it added a new dimension to my life, with my love and enjoyment of children."

Carol's dreams helped me accurately diagnose a problem she was having. In one of her dreams, there was a big lion residing in a back room of her house. "He roared louder and louder," she recalled. "Finally, when the noise got to me I opened the door and tossed a big hunk of cheese to the lion. Pretty soon the lion was purring like a pussycat and I got on with my work. Gladys asked me to interpret the dream. By this time I knew something about lining up the symbols. I told myself I had in the lion a potentially dangerous thing (illness) in my house (my body). But I could keep it under control, quiescent, by feeding it protein (the cheese). This helped Gladys to make the diagnosis of hypoglycemia—low blood sugar. All, as Gladys said, from the physician within me."

With her creative subconscious, Carol Brown had many prophetic dreams. Some were chilling and close to the bone, but since they came spontaneously, she reasoned they were meant to be. She was thankful for whatever guidance they gave her. She had been close to her mother, more so than most children. She had been an only child, with chronic asthma. The family had moved from the East, trying several climates before they settled in Arizona, where Carol pursued her career, married, and had her children.

"There was always a special bond between me and my parents, who had done so much for me, particularly between me and my mother, who watched over me like a mother hen. I had been thinking of my mother all this day and went to bed that night with her very much in my thoughts. She had been ill, and I was concerned. That night I dreamed my mother was in an airport, riding up an escalator. There was a crowd milling around and she seemed confused. I was standing on the other side of a glass partition, trying to get her attention. Again, I saw how bewildered she was. I shouted for her to follow the other people, telling her that she had wanted to make this journey for a long time. She would be fine. Then I woke with a start, a cold chill, a feeling of dread. And in a voice strangely my own asked aloud, 'Why is she taking this trip alone?' She usually traveled with my father. That night my mother died in California. In my sorrow I realized the dream was meant to prepare me for her 'moving on.' The ascending escalator was to let me know where she was bound. I was grateful to God for that dream. It softened the blow of losing someone who always put my life ahead of hers."

More often than not, my patients' dreams not only helped me with a diagnosis, they sometimes corrected my first impression. One patient of mine was continually catching cold, and quickly showing signs of fatigue. She looked like a normal, healthy young woman. I decided she had a vitamin C deficiency because of her susceptibility to colds. I was about to prescribe an increased intake of vitamin C when she told me of a dream she'd had the night before. She dreamt that she had left a store and was carrying home two bags of carrots when, from out of nowhere, a big lemon rolled off a roof and landed in one of her bags of carrots. She reached in, took out the lemon, and saw that it was rotten through and through. When I heard this I changed my diagnosis. Her dream told me that she needed more vitamin A—supplied by the carrots—and less vitamin C. I prescribed the A, and told her to eat carrots whenever so inclined. That's what the physician within her was telling us. And it worked.

I often tell patients that if they have a nagging problem, they should seek guidance from their dreams. They can ask God to help, then see what comes in the way of a dream. I mentioned this to a patient of mine who was undecided about having a tubal ligation. I had delivered three of her children, and now she was having trouble with the thought of a fourth. The children were so closely spaced, they were practically tumbling over one another.

I told her I couldn't make the decision for her. It was something only she and her husband could decide. "Why don't you try dreaming about it?" I suggested. Sometimes that was all that was necessary to get a person dreaming.

She meditated a few nights in a row, opening her subconscious, then placed a pencil and pad on a night table by her bed. Soon she had the following dream.

"My husband and I were riding down the freeway in a truck. On the back of the truck were three little Volkswagons (VWs). I had an idea these stood for my three children. Then as I was thinking about this in my dream, all of a sudden, from out of a side road hurtled another VW hellbent for destruction. It hit the side of our truck and turned everything upside down, including the truck and the three VWs."

She knew what that fourth VW signified, and she lost no time getting the tubal ligation. No way was that fourth VW coming into her family.

It's unfortunate so many people forget their dreams, even before they open their eyes in the morning. I tell patients to program themselves at bedtime for a night of dreams, to keep saying to themselves, "I will remember my dream." And you will remember.

However, if you don't take the time to write down the dream the moment you get up, chances are it will slide away. Once it's on paper you can go back and look at it, study it and analyze it.

For some people, taking vitamin B_6 at bedtime, about 100 milligrams, helps them remember their dreams. Medications, particularly sleeping pills, make it difficult to recall dreams. They block the creative alpha brain waves, as does an excess of alcohol and hard drugs.

Many dreams seem to manifest a past life experience. With the dreams of very small children, this can go beyond the scope of anything they could possibly remember in this life. Sometimes they wake up frightened and crying. Yet it's not till two or three years later, when they are able to talk, that they mention the strange places and languages they have seen and heard in their dreams.

In remembering dreams the important thing is the desire to remember. If you have not dreamt, or not remembered your dreams for a long time, it may take a while before your subconscious becomes aware that you are truly seeking a dream to resolve a serious problem. If you persist, you will begin to dream and know the answer. There's no way you can fool your subconscious mind.

I had long puzzled over the case of an attractive, otherwise normal young married woman who went into hysterics at the thought of becoming pregnant. Yet she expressed a desperate desire for a child. She had come to me only recently. She had been on the birth control pill for nine years, and was not yet 30.

"Why not give yourself a chance?" I suggested. "Stop the pill and see what happens. You say you want a child and would enjoy bringing it up. What can you lose?"

The woman shook herself. "It's these dreams I've been having. Nightmares. Ever since I was 14 years old."

I saw how difficult it was for her to deal with it. She was in a cold sweat and her hands trembled. It took her months to talk about it. The recurring nightmares were essentially the same. In these dreams she saw herself lying on the ground, her legs twisted together and her arms tied down. It was her feeling that she was pregnant and in labor. Her pain was intolerable. She woke up screaming for help in this dream within a dream, knowing there was nobody to help her, nobody to even untie her feet. She went through torment for hours, then woke up, just as she was about to die in the dream.

We talked the dream over after she had settled down a bit. I felt she was sincere in her desire for a child and was supported in this by her husband. She had toyed with the thought of a past life, and we discussed whether she had had a past experience where she died in childbirth. She was confused and didn't know what to believe. What she did know was that any thought of that terrible dream experience horrified her. We talked about what it would mean if she found herself pregnant in spite of taking the pill. In such a case, I pointed out, her higher self—the physician within—would have made the decision. Would she be able to accept it with composure? She nodded yes, knowing that the message would then be clear, and that the nightmares would end.

Some dreams have a way of coming true against all odds. A young couple I knew, with two children, had decided to limit their family so they could devote more time to living an idealistic life contributing to the betterment of humankind. They prayed and meditated, trying to find affirmation of their decision in their dreams. Meanwhile, the wife had worn an IUD—an intrauterine device—for five years.

Every year, as part of his job, the husband went overseas for a week of business conferences. He had many dreams, and one dream stood out. In this dream he saw a man in white robes. This man said, "Your wife is going to have another baby." The husband laughed in the dream and said, "That's not possible. She's wearing an IUD."

The man clothed in white held out his hand to the father. In his hand was an IUD. Here the dream ended.

When he came back to the States, the husband told his wife about the dream. They laughed and put it aside. The next spring he was scheduled to make the same trip, but due to other demands he was unable to leave the country and stayed home. That week, his wife became pregnant, even with the IUD. Both decided this was the physician within speaking. She carried the baby to term. I delivered the baby, first removing the IUD. In the labor room I reached across the delivery table to the patient's husband with the IUD in my hand. Recreating the dream I said, "This is yours, sir."

An Honor Roll

They use fear. And then they operate. I said good-bye.

—CORRINE LARSON

I had just been through a 12-hour day at the clinic and was a bit weary, but as I got to chatting with an associate about the physician within, my fatigue left me. I mentioned I'd like to go a little further than Doctor Schweitzer, and establish an honor roll of patients who brought the physician within to my doorstep by having that moment of illumination where they became the doctor.

"These," I said, "are my proudest moments. "You know, they don't need some strange and incurable disease to get on that roll. All it takes is sensitivity, openness, and honest-to-goodness guts."

"Is that all?" my colleague smiled.

"It happens," I said. "The physician within finds all kinds of ways."

Take Alice, for instance, a nomadic school teacher. Age-wise, you might say she was elderly—76 years old—but she moved around like a college coed. She was all over the place. She'd come to the office and never hold still long enough for me to examine her. She was always scooting off some place for an exotic adventure of one kind or another. She finally slowed down long enough to come into the clinic with a cancer that was so extensive it started in the cervix and extended to the rectum. She was bleeding. Since she never sat for a thorough examination, the cancer spread. But that didn't mean my friend Alice didn't have a physician within who was knocking on the door. She was just too busy to open the door. Later, however, it opened itself. I sent her to the surgeon, but he said he couldn't do any surgery until she had enough radiation to contain the cancer.

With two radiation treatments the cancer was contained sufficiently for the surgery to be done. But the day before she was scheduled for surgery Alice came into my office with disseminated herpes all over her body. She was a mess. She had an extensive infection and a temperature of 105 degrees. I thought, well she has decided somewhere inside her that this is her way out—out of the surgery and out of her life. This was the way she was going to check out. We put her in the hospital. For two weeks there were five of us working with her, trying to save her. The surgeon, the dermatologist, the infectious disease man, the internist and myself. I was beginning to think there was little else we could do. Then one day I went into her room and she was sitting up and the temperature was down. She was complaining about the food—always a good sign. I said to her, "Alice, what happened?"

There was the hint of a smile on her lips. And a look of uncertainty as though she was about to say something passing belief.

"I don't know how to say this," she began, "but yesterday, as though I was in my sleep, I heard soft bell-like music, not unlike a harp but different. I thought I must be dreaming. I had closed my eyes to visualize the music and then as I opened them I saw these little people, like munchkins or leprechauns, dancing on my bed. I was surrounded by them. They were no more than a foot or so tall. They were clad in homespun hats and shoes and long garments that were like cloaks or robes. They were all over my bed, working on me with their hands, without touching me, as if they were patching me up. I had an idea they were patching my aura, for their nimble little fingers kept weaving in and out around my head. They did this throughout the day. I suddenly found the fever leaving me. I felt composed, at peace, knowing everything was going to be all right. Then I dozed off to sleep. It was such a nice cozy feeling, drifting into unconsciousness. I thought, *if this is death, it isn't all that bad.* I don't know how long I slept. I woke up, refreshed, and the music started up again. I had to look around the room to make sure I wasn't in heaven with the angels, for the little men and women were still busy patching me up. Somehow, again, I knew they were working on my aura."

She was on the mend. Her temperature normal. She was restless, anxious to get going. She had been through the valley of death and it had no charms for her. She was her old self, aching to get out of the hospital.

Within a week or so we were able to send her home. In a couple of months we were able to perform surgery. I had a feeling she would come out of it better than ever. This was in the spring. In the fall we took a trip together to the Yucatan and Alice climbed every pyramid there was to climb. Afterwards she went to Northern California to run a goat farm. She was unpredictable, and that's how she liked it, one adventure after another, keeping her life moving, getting patched up every once in a while.

We talked about it. The physician within had crawled into her subconscious somehow, to get these little pixies to put her together. It was something I wouldn't have come up with. It was all within her. She did what she had to do to come out of it. I had a program ready for her, of visualization, diet and exercise. She saw no need for it. She had done what visualization she needed to do, got all the exercise anyone could handle climbing mountains and chasing after goats. And goat milk and yogurt were just what the physician within had ordered.

And what had touched off this physician? Her subconscious mind. She had come to the razor's edge and only then did she permit the physician within to do what had to be done to save her life.

There were others high on my Honor Roll. The Turkey Man, for instance, 72 years old, with an osteosarcoma of the shoulder. Part of the shoulder had been removed, but the cancer spread into his lungs. His chance of living more than a couple of months was slim. He didn't want to hear this and I didn't dwell on it.

A gutsy man, he had an active mind and meditated a lot. He had built his life on the earth as a farmer. He had a high regard for the Higher Power, having lived with all kinds of life on his farm. One night he had this dream that he was lying on the ground, pinned down by four wooden pegs. A small voice said, "These are the powers of the earth and you can't get up."

"You're wrong," he found himself saying, "I have 12 powers of the mind and I *will* get up." Being a man of purpose and intent he acted on this dream. He spent his winters in Arizona, then went up to Colorado and bought white turkeys. He spent the summer feeding his turkeys grasshoppers. He told the turkeys that the grasshoppers were cancer cells. And they, the turkeys, were his white disease-fighting cells. He worked the whole summer with that. He came back to Arizona the following winter, and back to Colorado in the summer, having now gone beyond his life expectancy. He got his white turkeys—the white blood cells—out again and fed them the grasshoppers. He was feeling fine but he may have had a premonition. That Thanksgiving he sold the turkeys. At Christmas time, in Arizona, he got the flu. He died in January. An autopsy showed no sign of cancer. He was ready to go.

Nobody could figure out what was wrong with Valdine, a young woman with a bad case of malaise and fatigue. There were no clues. She was known as the Mystery Patient. She had been sick from Christmas until April, hardly able to get around. I suggested a thorough massage, thinking it would increase her circulation, relax her, and put her body in touch with her mind. She was normally an active creative person. Even though she now looked like a prime candidate for the psychiatrist's couch, I saw positive signs: She had kept her sense of humor, even while feeling down. It showed something good was going on, ready to be touched off by the right spark.

After the massage, Valdine lay with eyes closed, warm and relaxed, her mind wandering where it pleased. She hadn't felt this good in months. As she opened her eyes an angel-like figure clad in a white robe floated into the room. The angel's silky blonde hair fell down to her shoulders and she spoke in a bell-like voice that reminded Valdine of the evening chimes. She thought of this angel as a *being,* feeling she had the benevolent aspect of an angel. The being's attention had been caught by a crystal pendant with a gold chain Valdine never removed in her waking hours. The cluster of crystals sparkled in the light. It was a prize possession, a gift from her husband the previous Christmas.

The being hovered over Valdine's bed. She would have reached out but the angel held up a slender hand and spoke with that musical voice. "That is a beautiful crystal necklace you have, but you wear it much too often. It shouldn't be worn all the time. Crystals produce a great deal of energy, confusing the energy created by your own body and mind. These energies get all tangled up, weakening your system. People know so little about crystals that they overdo it. Take the crystal off and put it in the sun. Let it clear itself, then put it back on, but not all the time or your energies will diminish. No more than a few hours a day. Do as we say."

Whatever it was, the power of suggestion or some higher power, my patient was immediately energized. She got off the table, slipped on a robe, then went into the hall and said to a therapist sitting outside the room, "Who was that person who just came in here?"

The therapist shook her head. "I've been sitting here right along. There was nobody."

I had seen this happen before. We don't give our bodies the credit we should for being able to communicate with our deeper being. Valdine's physician within knew what was bothering her, but it took this artful manipulation of the body to awaken the physician sufficiently to common the imagery of the subconscious mind. The patient's malaise vanished and she became again the active person she was before she received a crystal necklace for Christmas.

Occasionally, with children, I'm called on to make a decision so critical I pass it on to the parents. The mother had brought in an ailing boy I had delivered eight months before. She thought the baby was having a problem with his eye. I could see there was something radically wrong. I sent the mother to an ophthalmologist. He diagnosed a malignant melanoma on the eyeball, a rare disorder. From there they went to an eye clinic in Los Angeles.

Within 24 hours the mother called with a break in her voice. "I've had the worst news possible. The only thing they can do for my baby is take his eye out. I don't know what to do."

I thought about it a moment. It was a decision in good conscience I could not make. How could I go against two expert opinions in a situation where I was inclined to agree? But she needed to feel right about it, so I said, "Why don't you pray on it, make your best possible decision, then see what you get in the way of a dream?" I mentioned this had worked for me. "Make a prayer, saying to yourself, 'Okay, God, this is what I decided. That it's best to remove the baby's eye." Your dream will materialize, pro or con, if you pray hard enough and concentrate on remembering it. She dreamt that she was in a huge amphitheater with many other people. A giant of a man, some 20 feet tall, stepped over a wall and started eating the people. She was looking around for a way to escape when she spotted a crack in the wall. She slipped through the crack unnoticed and was free.

She had no trouble with the dream. She had worked out many of her dreams in the past. Obviously, the dream was a disaster. The crack in the wall was her clue. It was the only escape she had from a cancer that was eating people. She sighed and did what she had to do. Deep within herself she got an answer that none of us could give her. There was no way I would tell her to have her baby's eye removed. And there was no way she could make that decision without a deeper confirmation from the physician within. It was difficult but the choice had to be hers.

Nobody's quite the same, revealing anew how futile it is at times for a doctor to treat the disease instead of the person. One day, at different times, two women walked into my office with Lupus. It is a tough disease, and requires a lot of patience on the part of physician and patient. Lupus, as an autoimmune disorder, can place a heavy burden on the patient, since it feeds on the system. I had worked with one woman, Lynn, for many years. She still had her Lupus and she still had her problems. It was like we couldn't get anywhere with it. She had scaled down her life, and moved around like a semi-invalid.

I had puzzled over Lynn's case for some time, not understanding why she wasn't able to get on top of her problem until one day I went into the parking lot at lunchtime and saw her car. Her license plate said Lupus in big capital letters. I decided I'd have a talk with her. If a patient gets so identified with the disease process that they are the disease process, they have already lost considerable ground. Think deep into yourself, put the disease out of your mind, and let the physician within visualize a normal active life. More often than not, you will find new strength to carry on and do the things you want to do.

The other woman, Sherry, had been dealing with her Lupus for 10 years. She had awakened one morning in great pain and distress. Knowing the nature of her disease from our examination, she said to herself, "Here I am, lying in my bed in pain. Am I going to give in to it and spend the rest of my life this way?" It didn't take her long to come to a decision. There was a chair in her bedroom. She said to herself, "Pain, go sit in that chair and don't you ever get out." With great difficulty she got herself out of bed and moving around. Over a period of years, drawing on the forces within herself, she became functional enough to carry on with her profession. She was a college professor. In her classroom she keeps an empty chair. When the pain begins to bother her she sends it into that chair. I don't know how many of her students realize why that chair is sitting there empty, but her physician within knows. That's all the help and encouragement she needs.

A variety of therapists have been drawn to our clinic in Scottsdale to see for themselves how we're managing. They have a feeling we're doing something different, but what kind of magic is it? So what better way to get to know the answer than to become a patient with a problem that had been around for a while.

It was with curiosity as well as a need that Corrine Larson, a physical therapist for many years in Minnesota, knocked on our door. She had a small cyst under her arm. We talked about it. "It doesn't hurt," she said, "but I know it's there. I invariably ask when I visit a physician what I should do for it. It's a hard-walled cyst and it bothers me, but the doctors only shrug wisely."

I examined her and saw there were no cancerous implications, but it was best gone. We both agreed, "Rub some castor oil on it," I said. She was familiar with Edgar Cayce suggesting the cold-processed castor oil for so many different aberrations of the skin and body, but hadn't thought of applying it to herself.

Within two days the hard cystic walls softened, but then grew to be a large boil. Every day she put castor oil on it, and it grew larger. Alarmed, she went back to the clinic. I was out of the city. My daughter, Helene, lanced the boil. By this time it was huge.

"What happened?" Corrine asked. "Did I induce infection?"

Helene smiled. "No, the castor oil collected the infection from your body and brought it to a head. This is a normal process."

Corrine was looking for someone who could treat her in a natural way, with a compatible belief system she might learn by. She also had arthritis in both knees so bad she couldn't bend or unbend her legs. She meditated and visualized, clearing her knees of all impediments. A small voice told her she could change her standing in life. Standing. The word ended in her subconscious mind. She saw herself standing straight, without any strictures on her knees, no bone spurs and no arthritic joints. Everything as clean and clear with her knee joints as when she was a small girl jumping rope. Stand straight, the voice kept saying.

She had been sitting, meditating. Now she got up and with confidence stood straight and tall. She was healed. She had practiced what we taught and thought like we did. In her visualizations she reminded her subconscious mind what it was like to be without pain. The subconscious mind said, "I remember," and became connected, in a very gentle way, looking on to what the body remembered. Freedom from pain. People getting in touch with their inner selves. Journaling her feelings, moving to music and humming, viewing a piece of art, painting. Involving the mind and senses. Watching a great play or movie. Whenever you are in that timeless space of the subconscious the body is free to heal. This is one of the reasons visualizing of the healing process is so helpful. There is no end to what the subconscious mind can do when it is in place.

To some it all seemed too easy, too pat. So why the castor oil if the healing is in place? Corrine had no problem with it. "When you break it down, it's not all that simple. Castor oil has an affinity for pulling the poison. I believe so much this holistic physician can help me that my belief may also play a part along with her touch. Her presence, her interest calm you. When you hold tension in your body, you close off signals from the nerves, stifling the blood, nervous and nutritional systems. With tension your body has to struggle to get nourishment and is too busy fighting to get any healing done."

A long distance walker, Corrine teaches mind-connecting exercises such as yoga, tai chi and mentastics. These are exercises that keep you mobile and quiet the mind. Everything repressed comes to the surface, this leaves your mind free to be creative. Only a calm mind can be creative. The self feels a oneness, breathes deeply.

We have no boundaries. We make them for ourselves. A hundred and more years ago the province of the spirit was given to the church, the mind to the psychologists and the physical body to the medical practice. We got different activators working with the three divisions. It's time to put it together. We are one and this is the only way we heal.

Corrine has it down now.

"Our wholeness requires a unity of all our forces. We have to be our own physician. We gave ourselves to the specialists. And now with holistic medicine the patient is given the key to his own power. The body and mind remembers what it has never fully forgotten: how to heal itself with the force within."

Be Patient

*Give us grace and strength
to forbear and persevere . . .
courage and gaiety and
the quiet mind.*

—ROBERT LOUIS STEVENSON

Some patients hardly noticed the woman who sat just outside my office. She fit in like the furniture. She was 80 years old, and she drummed on an old typewriter like it was a piano. Her name was Grace Page. She was my secretary and conduit to the outside world, a voluntary worker. She had needed something to do—a purpose, a goal—and helped me to help those who suffered through many dark hours.

There was hardly an illness Grace hadn't struggled with: diabetes, arthritis, gangrene, shingles, tachycardia (irregular heart-
beat), neuropathy of the eyelid, chicken pox, circulatory
problems, and a massive heart attack, which had taken place in
my office. Grace Page was not one to inconvenience anyone if
she could help it. She's been my indispensable secretary since
I started taking care of her 30 years ago. She puts in a 25-hour
week, and is in constant communication with the outside
world. If it's about illness, she has the answer. She's been
through it, and she's constantly participating in the healing philosophy.

The tachycardia gave her a real problem. The heart beats so
fast that if you are under stress it can bring on a spasm. She went
to the hospital because of it, and enjoyed the rest. She has learned
patience, and how to outlast whatever disease she has had.

Her cardiologist had been surprised at the way she recovered
so quickly from the heart attack. I told her to visualize something that interested her, like the ocean. As she recalls:

"I lived in Hawaii for 10 years with my husband, so I visualized waves coming up on the beach and my sitting on the beach
as they rolled over me, so warm and soothing. With the gangrene in my toes I had visualized the blood flowing into my
feet—something I thought of myself. Gladys liked that, how I
caught on to the physician within. I had had circulation problems where the blood didn't flow as it should. My foot turned
blue so I knew the blood wasn't getting through. It took a month
for the gangrene to leave my toes and the skin color to become
normal. The blood vessels that were closed off stayed closed, but
new ancillary blood vessels developed and carried the blood to
the foot. It sounds kind of fantastic, but it happened. Listening to
soft music also helped. It relaxed every cell in my body."

Grace has had all kinds of visions, so vivid she felt she could
reach out and touch them. "I constantly sense my husband

around me," she says. "He once appeared in my dreams, saying he missed me and wanted me with him, but that it wasn't time for me to join him yet."

Grace was also the first person I used acupuncture on, to relieve her arthritis. That treatment brought on an internal awakening, in which Grace recognized the reality of her own healing force. "With the help of some tools from the outside I have become my own healer. I've faced life-threatening crises knowing I have the support and love of a husband I can still sense around me, and of Dr. Gladys. Her caring has much to do with my outlook. It keeps me up and at it, counting my blessings, knowing I have a lot of things to do yet on this planet. I've got a lot to stay around for. And a boss who needs me."

How would Grace Page have fared in the conventional healing process of traditional doctors with their bags of antibiotics and shots for everything from high blood pressure to arthritis, tachycardia and whatever else plagues humanity? Grace needed someone who cared and who knew the value of patience. One of the most important parts of therapy is allowing the healing to evolve the way the body tells it to. Conventional medicine, as opposed to holistic, tends to insist on a regimented healing process. If it isn't done in line with so-called normal medical practice, then it isn't right, and healing won't take place properly. The methodology appears at times to be more important than what's happening inside the patient's body. I've found we have to keep the patient comfortable, relaxed and confident, knowing they're cared for like a member of the family. We do a lot to make strangers feel at home, and we don't put limits on what we do. The younger people on our staff soon catch on.

Dr. Vickie Crowe was a recent addition to our crew. She soon showed how well she fit in. A young man with a splitting headache was one of her first patients. He had driven across the country, sleeping in his car at odd times, and he exhibited a lot of tension and stress. Vickie recognized immediately—because of the stiffness in his neck and his blood count—that it could be meningitis. There was no money for an MRI or a hospital. "He's just here," an aunt said. "He doesn't have work. This would have to come out of his mother's pocket and she doesn't have any money."

That didn't stop Vickie. She called the emergency room doctor who said if the young man was stuck in town they'd have to take care of him whether he had money or not. Vickie asked me to check him. He was obviously in serious condition.

We called the patient's mother, then the hospital, making all the arrangements. His mother drove him there. He received tests and antibiotics, and within 12 hours he was back with his mother, on the road to recovery. Vickie had quickly assumed her role as a holistic physician, incorporating the family in the healing process, and working with them. This interest gave the young man a boost in morale and the confidence he needed to heal rapidly. Meningitis was nothing to trifle with. Vickie's energy set up a positive vibration the young man could latch on to.

Sick people need support. They need to relax to get well, and they have to feel they're in the hands of people who care. Then the healing can take its natural course.

I have a feeling that conventional medicine, imbued with the psychology of sickness, overly belabors the weaknesses of the patient, and ignores the many strengths the sick have in areas not affected by the illness. Many patients are able to call on a vital life force deep within them, and mobilize healing energy to enhance their immune systems in the battle for life. I saw many remarkable instances of this in the face of devastating ailments.

One patient of mine was a real fighter. She was middle-aged, her husband had left her, and her business had failed. Yet she had overcome the incapacitating ravages of the dreaded multiple sclerosis (MS), amazing her neurologist as she recovered from a disease few recover from. She had lost the use of her right leg, hand and arm. She had no sense of equilibrium, and her nerve ends were deteriorating. "When the doctor stuck needles in me," she said, "I didn't even feel it."

One day she looked into the mirror, growled to herself, and said, "Nobody is going to do this to me. Nobody."

She knew something about meditation and visualization, and she reached for the physician within. It took a while for her subconscious, her inner self, to respond, but she kept needling it.

"I sent a message to every nerve and muscle in my body not to let MS get the best of it. I visualized a purifying process, beginning with the skin. I would visually scrub my skin clean, rubbing off the impurities inside and out. I mentally examined the bloodstream, cleansing the corpuscles, then washed off the muscle fibers. Visually, I stretched my muscles, hanging from a steel bar. Mentally, I attached sandbags to my feet to add that much more stretch. I coated my nerves with colored lights. Not knowing what color was most beneficial, I used every color in my imaginary rainbow."

In six weeks she noted an improvement in functioning. Her neurologist took new tests and they were negative. He took her off the hormone ACTH, warning her she would feel depressed until her system adjusted to the "high" the drug had given her. Going "cold turkey" was a withering experience. She went to a support group where others visualized along with her. She asked for new strength, meditating on a Higher Power. Almost immediately she felt a burst of energy and a wonderful feeling of lightness. She had no idea whether this was self-generated or the gift of others. Did it matter? She felt her depression lifting like a cloud before the wind. "I was a child of the universe, and the universe was taking care of its own."

Each time she went into her subconscious level she put herself on a pedestal. "I kept building myself up, countering the
blows that had toppled me from that pedestal in the first place."

This elevation of self-esteem was essential and was obviously
a motivating factor. She needed to believe in herself, to enforce
the physician within, to get the healing going. And this she
clearly did, with courage and perseverance.

She had gotten the negativity out of her life, something conventional physicians often overlook in the treatment of disease
rather than the whole person. We need to magnify the body's
virtues and minimize its faults, focusing on building up the
immune system and letting the weaker cells dwindle of themselves through a lack of attention.

People often ask me to name the one ingredient most lacking
in modern medicine. I can put it in one word: "patience."

And patience works both ways. Patients have to be patient
with their doctors, and their doctors have to be patient with
them. And they both must be patient—and persistent—with the
disease they face together. In the formative years of our holistic
association, our group realized the importance of patience in
healing, and not wanting to confuse the issue, we thought we
should call our patients "clients." But that didn't sound very caring. So we went back to "patients."

I've always been struck by what a wise Edgar Cayce had to
say about patience. "The more patience that is shown in self
toward others, the more patience will be shown by others to
self." This doesn't mean patience in the sense of submissiveness
or being quiet. It means an active and conscious awareness of
being patient in the healing process.

I once had a patient who was literally dying of cancer.
Her difficulty—frustrating both me, her physician, and the
physician within her—was not her apparent patience, but

her submissiveness. She had a husband who pushed her down and held her down. A kind word rarely came out of him. He made it clear that he had no sympathy for her. She didn't want to leave the hospital and go home because with the cancer he didn't want to touch her, as though she were unclean and the touch would contaminate him. He gave her food and walked away from her, but there was no involvement on his part in the healing. She had a dreadful feeling of being alone in her need, and she was so thoroughly submissive that there was little I could do to change things. I couldn't help thinking that her husband's impatience and her submissiveness could very well have had something to do with her illness. I never saw her again after she left the hospital, and that didn't surprise me. She had so little to live for.

Negativity in the home or in a doctor can be a killer. If a doctor says to a patient, "You've got cancer. You have six months to live," the body remembers this with its innate intelligence, whether the person thinks about it or not. On the other hand, if the physician can provide even a slight ray of hope, whether the patient consciously accepts it or not, the body, by the same token, can understand and grab hold of it. One of the worst things physicians can do is set themselves up as God and tell patients how much time they have left. What makes it worse, these physicians are often wrong. And even being right is hardly a victory.

I've heard adults of some distinction say that it's impatience—and discontent—that moves the world. That may be true, but it doesn't necessarily make it a better place.

Older people are more inclined to patience. Perhaps that's why they last as long as they do.

Joan Stamper was one of these longtime survivors. In her late 70s, she thought nothing of bicycling around town. She was impressive-looking too, still handsome, with the weather-beaten face of an outdoor woman. She looked healthy and capable.

Joan had been coming to me for eight months—as a doctor of last resort. She had been to a number of other doctors and none had been able to help her. At our clinic she was now getting help. She was out of pain, comfortable, and able once more to do the physical things she had stopped doing because of her illness.

I had delivered Joan's ninth and last baby 35 years before. We had not seen each other since, until her most recent doctor sent her to me. The diagnosis was scleroderma, a thickening of the connective tissues, an autoimmune disease in the arthritis family that feeds on itself. She quickly brought me up to date.

She had exercised regularly, doing yoga, standing on her head until three years ago, when she could no longer brace her wrists on the floor. She knew then that something was wrong. The search for a cure began.

"The first doctor said I was depressed. Of course I was depressed. Who wouldn't be? I wasn't bedridden, but I had no energy. I was living alone, frightened, in constant pain. I didn't know what was happening, and neither did anyone else. The pain was all over. The only places I didn't hurt were my head and feet. I had a feeling of tightness, difficulty in movement. I was getting progressively worse. This doctor said I needed Prozac, an antidepressant. How could the Prozac help what was disabling me? I decided not to go back. I frequently have an intuitive feeling about what is right for me.

"Then I went to an osteopath. I thought he might be more sensitive. He said I had a collagen disease and suggested I see a rheumatologist, who diagnosed scleroderma. He gave me pain pills but they didn't do much. Then he prescribed an anti-inflammatory drug, which anyone over 60 shouldn't take. Now I was getting impatient. They were giving me drugs that didn't help, so I started to read up on what I had. That was even more confusing. I don't normally complain, but after two years of this, I was getting very discouraged.

"Fortunately I had my faith to fall back on. I'm a Catholic. I get up every morning between five and six o'clock and go to mass. I'm a secular Franciscan, a person who follows the rules of St. Francis of Assisi in lay life. There is always something to do, someone to help. I think that's what kept me afloat those two years—keeping busy and communing with God. And talking to one of my children an hour a day was as important to me as getting legislation through congress.

"I was having trouble clenching my hands and this was a little unnerving. I could see the disease creeping in on me. I found yet another doctor. I don't know why I didn't think of Dr. Gladys. I had always thought of her as being so great, from the brief contact we had when I gave birth to my last child.

"I tried this new doctor briefly—another rheumatologist. When you're sick for so long without anyone helping, you'll poke into almost any door. This new rheumatologist was a nice man who listened, but he recommended a risky penicillin drug. You have to monitor your kidneys when you take that drug, and it sometimes does damage. I thought my kidneys were working fine. Why bother them? So then I went to a holistic doctor, a general practitioner. He suggested I see Dr. Gladys and talk over my problems with her.

"It may seem odd that I didn't think of Dr. Gladys myself. I guess I had put her in the 'baby department.' But she was the one who finally took charge."

I was happy to see Joan again. I gave her some exercises to do and some nutritional hints—cutting out red meat, eating more fresh fruits and vegetables. I encouraged regular massages and castor oil packs on her liver four times a week. I also got her back to exercising in moderation and her wrist action improved. She bicycled every day and swam in an outdoor pool in summer. Her daughter, a masseuse, massaged her every week. This helped to break up the hardened tissue from the scleroderma and get her lymphatic system moving. That in turn helped her fight the infection. But there was even more to do.

"Dr. Gladys told me to look within myself, both in mind and body. And I did. Today, I'm busy and active in my church and for my family. Recently I went to a friend's house to take her shopping and do some chores. She can't get around very well. She's having her hair done, while I'm visiting at the clinic. Tonight I will read, write letters, cook. I may even clean house. I am a loner. I don't mind it. I need to be alone at times to recharge.

"I am happy, relatively comfortable and active. I'm no longer depressed or discouraged. I found a doctor who has a C.D. degree. A Caring Doctor."

The Tiger Kitten

*You may house their
bodies but not their souls.
For their souls dwell in the
house of tomorrow.*

—KAHLIL GIBRAN

They were like so many other parents. They wanted a special child. They were young and strong—not vain, but proud of what they were and what they were capable of. As their family doctor and a dear friend, I watched and approved while they prepared for their baby: a healthy baby with a strong heart and a keen mind, whom they could school and guide as he or she—they didn't care which—went through the various wonderful stages of childhood into maturity.

They exercised, they kept a nutritious diet. They took massage and other treatments to keep in shape. They meditated and kept their minds active, maintaining a positive attitude. And they prayed for a *special* child. Pregnancy became a reality, and they continued with their positive approach for the physical and spiritual well-being of mother and child. Their minds were filled with love and concern for this special child, and it was very special to them. They were special, too.

Then came the big day and the child was born—a girl. They called her Tara. Their hearts were filled with joy.

The obstetrician held the baby in her arms for a moment, then handed her to the waiting mother, who smiled and caressed the child. The baby's eyes were closed, but they would open when it was time.

It was a normal pregnancy and a normal delivery. Nothing had gone wrong in the birthing. But something was not quite right. The child's movements, and her color were off. She was not a normal baby. It took nine months, ironically, for the doctors to confirm that little Tara had a rare chromosome disorder and a serious heart condition. Only three other children had been known to be so afflicted. None lived to be more than one year old.

I grieved for the parents and the child, wondering from my own deeply held convictions what had been in God's mind. There had to be a reason. There was always a reason, particularly when you believed in the continuity of life.

Kathy, the mother, also wondered. She blamed herself in a *mea culpa* to the doctor she cared about, and who cared about her: "I feel so torn inside, and guilty too, because I loved her so from the start. Yet I had a difficult time accepting the fact that she had chosen an imperfect body. I blamed myself at first, thinking it was something I did or didn't do during my pregnancy, but I woke up and realized that Tara's message was loud and clear: 'Hey, this has been my choice. You have no reason to feel guilty. I have chosen life with a disability in order to learn a lesson and gain added wisdom.'"

It was apparent from the beginning that something had gone awry. Right after the baby was born, the father, Darryl, was upset and went home to get some rest. He had stayed close to his wife through the birthing process, pulling for her, working with her, with all his energy and love. He was stretched out. He fell asleep and had a dream, a dream such as he never had before. In the dream he saw a scrawny-looking little tiger kitten with a cast on one leg. The kitten was going from one couple to the next, asking to be taken in. None of the different couples in the dream wanted her. No one wanted the responsibility. When the little waif of a tiger kitten came to Darryl and Kathy, they said, "We'll take care of you. We want you even if these other people don't." The dream continued, and Darryl and Kathy cared for the kitten, fed her and loved her. She grew up to be a sleek beautiful tiger because of their love. Although they knew in the dream that they couldn't contain or control her, they knew that she returned their love.

Waking from a fitful sleep, Darryl returned to the hospital to find there was a problem with the baby's hip. The pediatricians had put a cast on her leg, just like the tiger kitten had had. It was then that they knew they had a tiger in their family. But they would love her, and hopefully, things would turn out well.

Darryl and Kathy showered their affection on the little girl, who had a mind of her own. In addition to her physical handicaps, she was emotionally fragile. She wouldn't let anyone but her parents touch her, not even the babysitter. She had a beautiful smile that lit up her face, but she also scowled. Her love for her parents was manifest in her singular attachment. The parents knew they were living on the edge. As Tara passed her first birthday, her parents realized that she had stayed alive longer than any of the children with the same malformation.

When Tara was 16 months old, her mother had a dream about this very special child that seemed to foreshadow her uneasy connection with life.

"I dreamed that the three of us, my husband, Tara and myself, were living in a rectory. It seemed it was also our lake home. Then a fire broke out. I panicked and ran for the door when I suddenly remembered Tara. Charging into her room, I grabbed her from her crib and lovingly and carefully wrapped her in our big green blanket. Then I proceeded to kick out the window and we made it out safely."

The mother discussed the dream with me. I had the feeling the dream was saying that the child snatched out of the flames was carried out safely through a window that opened unto a new life. I mentioned this to her.

A year and more passed, and the mother had another dream. In this dream she had parked her car in a big parking ramp to go shopping. "Upon parking it, I changed my mind and wanted my car back *now*. I looked at the parking ticket to check the location of the car and it said: Tara Christine. When I asked the attendant if I could get my car now, she shook her head and said that she couldn't release the car for two hours. I turned away, disappointed, but thought, 'Well, I'll just go home and wait.'"

Again the mother came to me. I felt this dream was telling us that Tara would most certainly be released soon, but we'd have to wait.

Tara died a few hours later that same day. She was released, and Kathy was with her. Feeling uneasy, Kathy had gone into the child's room and found her tossing restlessly with a high fever. She bundled her into the green blanket of her dream and rushed off to the hospital, praying all the way. The little tiger kitten, she felt, had gone on to another dimension. She would never leave their hearts, never grow old. She would always be the same special child with a magnetic smile. Kathy and her husband had to dig deep into themselves to come to some understanding of why Tara had been born as she was, and then taken away so soon. She was two and a half years old when she died.

The mother had moments of illumination. "Death," she decided, "can have a positive side. It brings out our higher self and jars us into examining our relations with the people we care about. It makes us question our own purpose. What are we here for? Are we doing all we should to make this a better world for us and our children? Our children. Yes. Our children. For all people's children suddenly became our children in our hearts."

Kathy had an idea that in some strange way her little girl was aware of the impact she'd have on other people's lives. She continued to feel the child's presence. It permeated the space she had occupied. She was missed, terribly, but not mourned. They knew she was safe now.

"I never thought I'd be able to handle death the way I have," Kathy later told me. "The universal laws do work. What you generate does return to you. Our emptiness has been filled with beautiful memories. When sadness steals in we replace it with the thought that Tara is no longer limited by her physical body. We are lonesome for her, but our prevalent feelings are peace, joy, happiness and a love that knows no time or place."

I was touched by something Kathy later wrote me in a letter: "Another good thing that has come about is my opportunity to share these meaningful thoughts and feelings. It helps to get my thoughts down in writing in order to sort out all of my feelings at this time. I've kept a lot inside and now I'm ready to share. It's our opportunity to help others deal with similar tragedies in their lives in a more positive and meaningful way."

Painting a Picture of Health

This was my last chance to keep out of a wheelchair.

—Barbara Miller

A line had formed after I finished my talk and began taking questions. I had just given a lecture at a Wellness Conference in Potomac, Maryland. For some reason my eye had picked out the pallid figure of a woman who had been inching her way forward in obvious pain, dragging one leg after the other. I could see her gritting her teeth, each step a labor of Hercules. I had been speaking about the power of the individuals to heal themselves, to find the physician within. I could see from the long line that my talk had made an impression on people who wanted to know more about this novel idea.

My eye kept note of the woman with the faltering gait even as I was taking questions. She seemed shy, unsure of herself, something a chronic illness will do to almost anyone. As she finally got to me, she looked around, noting the others pressing behind her. I saw her frown, and I thought for a moment that she was going to give up her place. In a mild voice she said she was sorry to intrude. Our eyes connected, and I had a feeling that this pasty-faced woman with the tired eyes had a dire need of me—a very special need. She asked if I could give her my card. I gave it to her, squeezed her hand and said I would like to hear from her. She thanked me and moved off with a man her own age—they were in their 40s—who I took for her husband. She looked back once. I caught her look and nodded. She needed all the encouragement I could give her. She was a sick woman, not quite at the edge.

It wasn't long before her husband called. She had given him my card. He came to the point, and I liked that. He described her illness, a serious back problem she had had almost from the day she took her first step. It was more an ailment than a disease—and about as hard to help as it was to spell: spondylolisthesis. I'd treated some patients with it in the Arizona clinic.

Her name was Barbara Miller and her husband's name was Richard. He was a successful businessman and motivator, and I could tell that he dearly loved his wife. He would do whatever he could for her.

"Can you help Barbara?" he said.

"I cannot promise anything," I said. "I have been able to help some people with it. But some I cannot help."

I suggested he bring Barbara out to our clinic and we would see what we could do.

He seemed pleased that I knew something about the problem, because it was not that common. It came about when a part of the fifth lumbar in the mid-back region, unformed from birth, slipped forward, putting pressure on the first sacral (pelvic) vertebra when the person walked. There was no way Barbara could get around without suffering agonizing pain.

Since I had some experience with the condition, they decided to come out to Scottsdale. Her husband had long before ruled out surgery. I assured him this was not a consideration. Barbara had weathered the trip well and seemed more settled and relaxed. We went over the difficulties she'd had in trying to find relief. It had been a nightmare. A professional painter, she had already given up her career. She had trouble walking or driving to a neighborhood store for groceries. She had become a semi-invalid and feared the worst—complete immobility and becoming a prisoner in her own home. She had been active before, working over the pain. That meant something to me, as her doctor. She was trying, she had desire, and that was half the battle. I could also sense her anger as she went into her medical history. Anger could be an incentive too.

"It was frightening," she said, "like I could lose the use of my legs forever. What next, my arms? And then the wheelchair? That's what the doctors saw for me."

Pounding on many doors she had become something of an authority on doctors. She had come to this conclusion: "It's very difficult to get the truth from any doctor who cannot cure you. They don't have much in their training to deal with anything chronic. And they don't like saying, 'Yes, you'll be in a wheelchair before long,' so they'll look off and say, 'Not this year.' That's their message of hope for the day."

She had been to arthritis and back specialists, osteopaths, chiropractors, orthopedists. She eventually developed a secondary arthritis, which added to the already unbearable pain. Her body had quivered from the nerve damage to a point where she'd wake up in the night with a vomiting spell. So violent were the spasms, she thought she would die. And she was almost relieved at the thought.

As I looked at her, I saw a new fire in her eye and a square jaw that bespoke an iron resolve. I thought we could help her, with her help. In the beginning she would be battling uphill much of the time. It would take a lot of effort on her part. I had made this clear before they traveled to Arizona, and I had mentioned the physician within. She needed to establish this link to the healing process. She also needed to maintain a rigid discipline in diet, exercise, massage therapy, and, most importantly, visualize the steps by which she would become well. None of this daunted her. She had some physical therapy that seemed to ease the pain. But something new developed that bothered her and her husband, something they hadn't counted on: the weather. We were in the midst of a typical Arizona desert summer, featuring 100-plus-degree days. It would pass, and there was always air conditioning, but both Barbara and her husband were concerned that the hot, dry climate might rob her of what little energy she could muster. They decided to go back east and give the move more thought, as it would mean taking a house and changing their lifestyle. I did nothing to influence her decision. It was all up to her. Any improvement would require a total commitment on her part. We said our goodbyes, but I had a feeling they would be back.

Back home, when the pain got too severe, she consulted an orthopedic surgeon. He convinced her—inadvertently—that she should go back to Arizona. A deepening arthritis had made it difficult for her to bend forward or backward. Her muscles were like steel cables, and she was pulling both legs after her. She couldn't sit comfortably in a chair. She told the surgeon that she couldn't sit, stand or walk without this severe pain.

He smiled. "Well, you should be in bed. When you get up in the morning and the pain is so intense that you don't feel well, you should spend the day in bed with your legs up on pillows."

She thought to herself, "This wasn't what my life was supposed to be about. I am a wife and a mother—with a grown daughter—and a professional artist with a compulsive desire to paint, whose career is on hold. How can I paint when he is telling me I can't even go to the store and buy a quart of milk?"

"I might as well be a cripple," she told the surgeon, "for all the good I'm doing myself or anyone else."

As the surgeon shrugged, her husband mentioned that she had seemed to improve after a few treatments at the Scottsdale clinic.

The surgeon waved that off. "It's the dry climate," he said, "not the treatment."

On the spot Barbara made her decision. "I decided I would be going back to Scottsdale and stay the course with a doctor who had me feeling I had a physician within who could help me."

Back in Arizona, Barbara plunged into her recovery. The preliminary diagnosis of a congenital malformation was confirmed during her treatments. There were osteopathic manipulations to make her spine more supple, deep massage to awaken the sleeping cells in her body, and acuscope (electronic acupuncture) to help control the pain. We also used biofeedback, with a machine that told both Barbara and the therapist when and how she had gotten into the healing alpha brain waves. This way she could repeat the process at will anytime she wanted, and she soon found she could send healing energy into any part of her body.

But Barbara was tiring, moving too fast. She wanted to do everything. We slowed her down.

By this time, she had reduced her pain by visualizing herself soaking in a hot tub, or relaxing in the warm ocean surf, or, ironically, sunbathing in the Arizona summer. Her subconscious mind, linked to the innate intelligence of every cell, was a natural conduit to her healing process. She pictured herself as stronger, more active, moving about briskly, playing tennis.

There were positive changes in her mobility and outlook. She no longer saw herself as a sick person, but as a well person, with correctable physical problems.

She had a good idea now of what she could accomplish, so it was time to give her body and mind a rest before she moved on to her next phase of healing. It was as if the physician within was saying "ease off for a while." During this rest period, Barbara began to realize how she had participated in her own illness by practicing denial.

"I was silent when I should have been speaking up to maintain my health. Women too often practice denial. The Maryland weather wasn't good for what I had. I needed a warmer, drier climate. I was also climbing stairs, the last thing I should have done. It threw my vertebra further out of joint. Because of the constant pain I was too much into self-pity. Without realizing it, I had given up. I stopped thinking about the positive, creative life I should have had, and instead focused on every little pain I had. I realized during this rest period that I had to reconstruct my thinking—and not about my body, or even about getting well. Instead, I had to figure out how I could become more productive and help the people around me. To do that I had to look ahead, beyond my pain, and not live in the shadowy image of an aging woman struggling with the minutiae in her life. I need to look ahead to a life of service."

Developing this inner consciousness was an important part of Barbara's healing. The physician within had come of age.

I told her, "You can do whatever you want. Just think hard about it and see yourself doing it. Concentrate. And do it with a sense of humor—you don't have to be perfect. Be able to laugh at yourself if you stumble a little. Don't be afraid of trying an exercise or a flight of mind or fantasy. Banish fear from your consciousness. It's an adversary always lurking, ready to pounce. Be brave and expectant—of the best."

It was important for her to get back to her painting, and we worked on imagery, through her dreams. In this way she would get to know more about her inner self. Her face lit up when I mentioned a dream journal. As an artist she had a vivid imagination. She was still feeling pain, and the thought of dreaming this away intrigued her. She went to sleep with a dream journal on her night table. Her dreams soon confirmed what she had been thinking for some time: something in her life had to be changed. Night after night she dreamed of a setting sun that looked like an eye with a tear in it. The setting sun represented the dying day in her mind. Was it weeping for her? She laughed, and then visualized the rising sun—a new day.

Dreams played an important part in Barbara's physical recovery. She soon discovered that the mind and body are one. In her dreams she visualized healing solar rays flowing into her lower back. She was able to recapture this dream in the alpha state with the biofeedback machine, producing with her subconscious mind the same healing energy with a significant rise in temperature to the affected lower back region.

She found herself getting muscle strength back in her legs, and feeling returned in prickling waves to her feet, which some doctors had thought might become gangrenous. New cells were starting to regenerate where the nerves were damaged, something that had been thought medically impossible.

The biggest change was in Barbara's mental outlook. I told her that to stay healthy she would have to live simply, husband her strength and not try to prove that she could do anything that anyone with a normal back could do. She and her husband moved into a new one-story ranch home in Scottsdale—no more steps to climb. She found she could drive again, if she didn't drive a long distance. But in time she found she could drive to the airport, which was some distance, and pick up friends. Her confidence was coming back.

As another part of her treatment, I liked to get Barbara talking about her healing herself. It helped confirm the healing process in her mind and revealed some special insights. As Barbara explains, "Soon you start knowing things you should be doing for yourself. You become aware of warning pains when doing an exercise that may further displace the weakened vertebra. You know this physician within is guiding you.

"I was also dealing more with my dreams. There was one dream that really threw me. I had no trouble interpreting it. You get to know in your meditations that the symbols are what you make of them, and that the dream is talking to you. In this one dream, I saw myself in a beautiful apartment. It was light and airy, elegantly furnished. Music was playing and a party was in progress. I was singing the lyrics from *New York, New York*, about being on top of the heap.

"My doctor came into my dream and told me that I had been on the third floor, but now I was in the penthouse. I said, 'Does that mean I'm not going to improve?' He shook his head. 'No. Just enjoy where you are.'"

I'd told Barbara that any apartment dreams would most likely represent her spine. The different stories were like the many vertebrae in her spinal column. She had reached the peak—the penthouse—the top of the heap. You couldn't get any higher without flying. I encouraged Barbara to keep up with her dream journal and to tell herself at bedtime that she would remember whatever she dreamt.

Barbara had also prayed most of her life, visualizing Jesus and the saints, so it was no surprise that her newly expanded subconscious was brimming with dreams of angels. Her angels appeared in forms that were vague at times, and androgynous, neither male nor female. But their messages, which she somehow picked up on spontaneously and without conscious thought, were communicated to the canvases she was now beginning to work on with her increased mobility. She painted dark, mysterious figures which on close examination became the visionary angels of her dreams.

Getting back to her easel had much to do with quickening Barbara's recovery. It had been a while since she had put away her brush and palette, but now she felt the exhilaration and joy of a redeemed artist in command of this subconscious part of herself. And painting utilized the same alpha brain waves that were also involved in the healing process. She was literally healing herself as she painted. Barbara had once been to Jerusalem, to the Wailing Wall where Jews had prayed for 3,000 years, and now she was moved to recreate the wall on canvas. It was a soul-lifting experience such as she had never known before. She seemed suddenly to be at one with the Creator, and his creation.

"In waves and waves of energy coming through the stones, God was speaking to me—and yet there was silence. I was overwhelmed with the knowledge of how much God loves us. I prayed for my family, for my daughter's unborn child. 'May she be all you want her to be, God. Thank you for my life in your Universe.'"

It was a mystery that left her exalted, ready to mingle with the angels who had become so much of her subconscious life, and so helped her that she felt she would never again be burdened with anything she couldn't handle. It was something she would have to keep working on, but the effort—the painting, the creating, the loving and being loved, communicating with the physician within her—was part of what God had spoken in the silence of the wall.

"I talk with the angels and they help me to be aware of some things I do that are slowing my growth. Although I don't hear what they say, the words are engraved on my mind as clearly as anything can be. They tell me when I have worked too long in my garden, run too long on my treadmill. I think of them as a manifestation of God's energy. I paint better, with greater facility and heart, because they come through the paintings.

It was a challenge, with never a thought of dropping out. Not while she had her dreams, and her painting, the angels, and the physician within. With God in the "wings." The word came to her without her thinking about it. She smiled.

"It's never easy. But nobody promised me a rose garden. I have times when I'm discouraged and tell the angels I'm stressed out in a material world, spinning myself too fast, not keeping myself centered, forgetting in my enthusiasm at my improvement that my body still becomes tired after being driven at a fast pace for three or four hours. I ask questions of the angels and they sometimes answer them in my dreams. I have very active dreams, and usually write them down. I suppose these angels might be called my guides, the physicians within. They don't have wings, but they do have the force to change my perception of things: to hold on to and give me strength, to help me."

With all that Barbara had been through, her paintings took on a new tone, a surrealism that depicted the workings of the subconscious mind, and a mind that had worked for her in conducting her own healings. I noted the difference in her work, as did the critics, compared to what she had done 20 and 30 years before. The transition was remarkable and revealing. In the earlier pictures there was a harshness and starkness: a naked contorted figure of a woman with her face shielded by an arm, the suffering plainly etched in the monolithic background and the severity of her posture. The body was balanced on what looked to be a huge block of stone. It could have been any woman suffering, maltreated, despondent, beaten down, stricken by an uncaring world. It had strength—mirroring the futility and hopelessness of a woman overwhelmed and trampled underfoot by life.

Was this how she had seen herself then? As her doctor and her mentor, it would have been disingenuous to ask.

Her new paintings, reflecting the artist and physician within, were a mélange of color and mystique with a myriad of mysterious figures, some of them angels, poking their obscure faces out of the hidden folds of brilliant color. As with true impressionistic art, different people saw different things in her work. One critic observed, "It all comes together, in many images: creation, angels, mother and child, figures from the Bible, tiny voices of the inner self."

That inner self was crucial. Barbara Miller had not only healed her body but her spirit and mind.

Barbara also continued dreaming and interpreting those dreams in light of her healing. Two years after first coming to the Scottsdale clinic, she dreamed of an intensely blue sky. Birds holding a long ribbon and bows in their beaks were flying across the sky. Voices were saying, "White doves are sailing. White doves are sai-i-ling. White doves are sailing ho-o-ome to me."

Barbara was now a dream expert, and the symbolism seemed clear to her. The doves were symbols of peace, love and the holy spirit. They were coming to her home to help her. The emphasis was in the words *sailing* and *home*. So Barbara figured it would take a while yet. But fundamentally it was a dream of encouragement, supporting the efforts she was making. She felt reassured.

A few months later she had a dream she puzzled over for a while. She was wearing black, high-heeled shoes with black nylons, rolled down to the ankles. A black snake was wrapping itself around her feet. She woke up in a cold sweat. She hated snakes. It took her a while to work this dream out. Black stood for a dark truth, in the shadows and therefore unrecognized. Obviously, the shoes would be difficult to walk around in comfortably, and with the snake nipping at her bare ankles, she was not to do too much walking while encumbered. In other words, the message was: don't overextend yourself. The snake, which gave her the shivers even thinking about it, was a warning: Back away. Don't knock yourself out.

Barbara has learned to respect the voice within, a voice that is quiet but insistent. "For the first time I feel as if I can handle whatever I have to. I can deal with my pain and my changing horizons. My morning prayer has become the same prayer I say before starting my painting each day:

"Dear God, let me join with Creation in living a life where I go beyond the pain and live a fuller life. I thank you for what you have given me: my friends, my family, my angels and my dreams. And thank you for the physician within that I have learned to trust, and for the will to stand on my own two feet, with my palette and brush firmly in my hand and a prayer on my lips."

17

Getting off the
Merry-Go-Round

No coward soul is mine,
I see Heaven's glories shine,
And faith shines equal,
Arming me from fear.

—EMILY BRONTË

All her life Carol Brown's been a mind dragging a body around after her.

She is a brilliant writer and newspaper reporter, with a wall full of awards. Her eyes are bright and perceptive, and like a few reporters I've known, she has a way of anticipating a question, and then running away with the answer. She is slight in stature and body but there is a wiriness, a toughness, that says she has borne and could bear whatever she has to.

She has a fragile body that looks like it might blow away in a stiff wind. She weighs about 90 pounds soaking wet, but she has an incredible spirit and drive. Last year alone she got five awards, some national, including Woman Writer of the Year from the National Federation of Press Women. She keeps traveling, searching, wanting to know more and tell more. A year and a half ago she went to Africa with a group of reporters. I was concerned because that's a pretty big trip for someone with all the problems she's had—chronic asthma, lots of lung and bronchial complications that she was born with. But Carol doesn't stop at anything. She sees something to be done and she says, "Come on body, we've got something to do." She has two sons, now grown, but as tiny as she is, she nursed both of them as infants while holding down a couple of jobs. When she decides she's going to do something, her body had better cooperate because she's going to do it.

She's a perfect example of the ongoing healing process because with Carol Brown, like so many of the patients I work with, it's not a matter of curing a disease, but of healing body and mind. The kind of problem Carol has will probably stay with her until she dies. But this problem—that might kill anybody else—will not kill Carol.

It's also not a matter of having to "live with it." Carol doesn't think that way. She has chronic lung problems, a scoliosis or curvature of her spine, and her whole physical system is very fragile. The reason I didn't want her to go to Africa was because she could get an infection and it would be pretty hard on her. But Carol went anyway, and she didn't get any infection.

As a child, Carol's family shielded her. Now when she does get sick, she does the things she needs to do and she just gets over it. If she needs an antibiotic, she'll take it, but she'll also use glycothymoline (to alkalinize mucous), camphoderm (to stimulate the lymphatics), and oaken brandy keg fumes (to assist breathing). All these different Cayce modalities help her get over her respiratory problems, and she also uses castor oil packs on her liver.

I have often wondered about the various dimensions of courage. Who is the braver—the gutsier, the one who knows no fear, the classic hero or heroine who plunges into danger without a tremor, or the one who wavered with just a twitch in the pit of the stomach?

I had an idea Carol Brown would know.

"So," Carol says, her dark eyes sparkling, "how did I conquer my fear?" She smiles. "I'm not sure which fear you're referring to. I had so many. But, generally, I've been able to put aside my fears through a combination of prayer and positive self-talk. I remember talking myself through scary, painful situations as a child. If I had to have a shot or any mysterious medical procedure, I'd say to myself, 'It will be over in the blink of an eye.' I also had things to do in my mind if, for example, a stranger followed me, like running faster than he could. My parents were Jewish, but my mother converted and she had a lot of Catholic friends. Our family didn't go to temple or church much, largely due to my dad traveling for his business, and me being down with my asthma half the time as a kid. But I always said my prayers and hoped God was looking after us. I sort of developed my own relationship with God as a friend and protector. I figured that he didn't much mind if I talked to him in the desert or in a dark alley. I sensed he could hear me anywhere. And I decided anyway, even as a kid, that it was more important that I hear him and what he had to say to all of us.

"I figured that God helps those who help themselves. So it was up to me to do a lot of the work. I remember being lost on a street corner in the city when I was six or seven. My mother had got separated in the street traffic. All the cars whizzed by. I was standing there, crying, and no one paid any attention. Right then I understood that everyone was busy with their own lives and if

I needed help I would have to ask God to help me—and then search for a friendly-looking person. Later in life, I got acquainted with the positive thinking of Norman Vincent Peale, and I would save quotations of his that inspired me whenever I faced a scary situation. The worst thing I could do was to give in to my fears.

"I may have been most fearful when raising two teenagers. I'd stay up at night, waiting, when they'd just learned to drive. I soon learned that one cannot operate from a place of fear. It paralyzes the mind, body and spirit. When I find myself in a bind today I say a quiet prayer, using some visualization techniques, like seeing twin doves of peace, and letting God lead me to the best solution.

"Everything came together for me, luckily, when Gladys told me about the physician within some 30 years ago. She taught me to listen to the signals my body was giving me, to meditate, slow down and take time for myself so my health would improve and I could do more. She taught me some positive affirmation techniques, visualizing myself in a white light or doing deep yoga breathing. It was all new to me. My parents, bless them, didn't know anything about holistic medicine (except for using chicken soup for colds). They came from a generation that totally relied on antibiotics, steroids and surgery. Gladys gave me the mind-body-spirit connection. I was hungry for something more, fed up with so many physicians' quick-fix approaches.

"When I became pregnant, I wanted to do natural childbirth and nurse my baby. I guess God and my unborn child led me to Gladys. We started talking about things like universal laws, mind healing things I'd been working at intuitively. She gave me the key—or maybe she just told me what pocket it was hiding in—to the bigger picture, the whole universe and the whole person. This encouraged me to become patient, willing to experiment with treatments of a holistic nature. Fortunately, I had an open-minded husband who gave me the support I needed.

"My family made sacrifices for me, moving from New York to Arizona. Three-quarters of their income was spent on medical bills for me. They were even investigated by the IRS, who couldn't understand how they could survive paying such high medical bills for this kid. But they did it, barely. As a kid I got shots to open my bronchial tubes. I was once given 48 hours to live. The doctors told my mom to take me to Hawaii or Prescott, Arizona, where the altitude is 5,000 feet. She got on a night train for Arizona.

"Later, when it got so I couldn't breathe in school, my mother had me whip out a note that said, 'Don't panic, I'm having an asthma attack. The school nurse has my medicine. Call her immediately.' The teacher would get all upset and the kids would start yelling. That would scare me and make me worse. I had allergies too. I couldn't drink cold milk or go out at night. There could be no stuffed animals or rugs. I couldn't have a dog or cat because of my allergies. Sometimes a kindly doctor would say, within my hearing, 'She may grow out of it.' Now as I look back, I can see it grew out of me.

"I'd run short of oxygen. The doctors told my mother not to do anything until I turned blue. When there was no adrenaline available she'd whack me hard so I'd start crying, and that would raise the adrenaline level in my body. I was about eight or nine then, growing up. She would grab my hands to see if my fingernails were turning blue. She wouldn't let me wear nail polish for that reason. But she was always upbeat. She'd say, 'You can do anything you want with your life. You just got to want it enough.' She said this even though she was practically a basket case from handling me. All I saw was doctors, and one I particularly remember. Gladys had a good laugh when I told her about it. This doctor told me to eat lamb chops three times a day for four months. I'd probably be dead now if lamb chops hadn't been so expensive."

Carol had a sense of humor that was "required healing." She was too busy with her traveling and writing to find time to brood over what might have been or should have been. She had reason to believe the good Lord was watching over her. She had asked for strength as she grew into her teens and beyond, and he had given her challenges. In college she had a roommate who also had asthma. She was from Texas and six feet tall, head and shoulders over the five-foot-two Carol.

"We called her Tex because she was from Texas. She used the same medicine I used for my asthma. We pledged different sororities, and she moved to an upstairs room in the same dormitory. I worried about her. We were like sisters. I said, 'If you ever run out of epinephrine, just send one of your sorority sisters down to me. I'll keep some special for you.'

"A year later she had an asthma attack in the middle of the night. She was choking for air and she panicked. Instead of sending for somebody, and obsessed by fear, she ran down two flights of stairs and right through the plate glass doors at the bottom. She had a heart attack and died at 19."

Carol did some deep thinking about it. It turned her life around to some extent, because it made her dig into herself to understand what had happened to this young woman she had cared about, and who had shared her illness and what went with it. She had been wonderfully alive one moment, dead a few moments later.

"When the campus medics arrived, they said she died of an asthma attack. It was a shock to all of us college kids—that somebody that young had died. I thought about my own years of fighting asthma, and I knew intuitively that she hadn't died of an asthma attack—she had died of fear. Her fear caused her to close up, and that triggered the heart attack. Some of the kids said, 'Gosh, you've got the same asthma. Aren't you afraid you're going to drop dead?'"

Carol remembers shaking her head and saying, "'No, you stay calm and handle it.'

"It hit me then, for the first time in my life, that what you do with your mind may make all the difference between life and death. It was a tragedy that didn't have to happen."

Carol learned from it and it may have saved her life. One day she was driving home from the Phoenix paper she worked for. It was a hot humid day on the desert, the temperature passed the 100 mark. The air was heavy and close for an average person, but it was horrific for an asthmatic. It was getting difficult for Carol to breathe. She looked around for her medicine, and then realized she had changed purses—and her medicine was in the other purse. She was in a traffic jam and she had nowhere to go. "I was having trouble breathing," Carol remembers. "I looked in the purse again—no medicine. For an instant I started to panic, then I thought of the friend I had lost when she panicked. My mood changed and I lightened up. I thought, what would they put on my tombstone: 'Died in a Traffic Jam'? And I said to myself, 'No way. Start using your old bean. Keep your cool.' I looked out the windows and the cars still weren't moving. It looked like they were never going to move. 'You're okay,' I said to myself. 'You'll be home soon. Breathe deeply. Think about the ocean and the mountains. What would Gladys have you do? Take your mind off this traffic jam—it's been like this before, and it has to end. People have to get home and have their dinners and get to bed so they can get up in the morning and get in another jam.'" The thought amused her and she started to laugh.

"I knew it would be all right then. My breathing kept getting better. I knew enough to sit still and be quiet, just breathing, like a yogi. If I opened the car door and yelled for help, what could anybody do? They were stuck in the same jam. I was there for an hour or so, and I couldn't afford to be frightened. By the time I got home, I didn't need any medicine. I had relaxed myself

with my deep, even breathing, and with a little humor. I had
banished fear and the threat of an attack with my mind. I thought
again of Gladys, and how she had turned around my thinking."

Self-discipline and patience also contributed to Carol's healing,
and self-discipline, like charity, should begin at home.

"My son as a boy got painful earaches," Carol told me, "from
being out in a heavy wind. I had warned him about this. I could
have given him a pill that would have eased the pain, but I delib-
erately withheld it. We were all at dinner, and my husband got
upset. 'Why don't you give the boy the pill? Can't you see he's
in pain?'"

The boy was six or seven at the time. "It was his choice,"
Carol said. "He chose to go out and play in the wind, breathing
in the dust and pollen. It gave him a sinus headache and an ear-
ache, as he had been told it would."

She turned to the boy. He was rubbing his eyes. It was almost
enough to make the mother in Carol relent. But she had not
fashioned her life with "almosts." She said to her son, "The next
time you want to go out and play in the wind, think about how
you're feeling now. I'm not giving you a pill to make it go away.
If you had stayed inside, you wouldn't be needing it."

This was a lesson that might stand him in good stead one day.
A few days later, Carol overheard her son telling his friends that
he couldn't go out and play because the wind made him sick.
He was learning to consider what was best for him. And what
was best, Carol thought, was that he was learning to think—a
quality that would serve him well the rest of his life.

"I wanted him to know he was in charge and had a choice.
If he wanted to put up with the pain, he could go out in the
wind. But he'd have to pay the price."

Carol had come down with pneumonia four times in five
years from doing too much. She was active in her children's

school, worked with the newspaper, wrote for magazines, and was busy with her photography. And she managed a household. As Carol thought about it, she realized she wasn't measuring up to her own belief system of "easy does it."

"This winter," she announced to me, "I'm not going to have pneumonia." I smiled. "Well, now that it got your attention, maybe you can do something about it, and connect up with the physician within."

She upped her intake of vitamin C and cut down on her school time and on her stress levels. "Things had been ganging up on me and I needed a breather—literally. I used an Edgar Cayce remedy: breathing in apple brandy fumes from a charred oak keg twice a day. It helps repair inflamed lung tissue and opens up the bronchial tubes, forestalling colds and infections."

I had advised this treatment for many others, including a friend's son, a six-year-old boy with a deadly asthmatic condition. His malady had been described as hopeless by doctors, but with the Cayce remedy, he was breathing normally in a few weeks.

I also suspected that Carol had hypoglycemia. She was nursing one of her children, working overtime, tired all the time and going on chocolate binges. Diabetes was calling. "Why," I suggested, "don't you come in for a glucose tolerance test? In the meantime, start recording your dreams."

Carol came up with the dream about tossing a hunk of cheese at an angry lion. That protein, helpful for low blood sugar, quieted the lion. And Carol's glucose test showed her blood sugar was significantly abnormal.

Her inner connection was already telling her she'd better cut down on sugars and build up her immune system. She had a series of vitamin B_{12} shots, and massages to help her circulation and awaken the affected cells. She didn't let fear get woven into her system. "It was always a battle between me and fear. You couldn't let fear win the battle, or it would go on and win the war."

Once Carol was trapped in a dust storm, 30 miles outside Phoenix. She had to be in two places at the same time—interviewing a singer for her Phoenix paper and covering a sheep drive for a magazine. Now she was stuck in a storm.

"I'm in a dust storm," she thought to herself, "and I don't have my medicine, and I'm going to be sick because of this." As soon as this went through her mind she thought of her inner connection and said to herself, "Don't say that. You can't afford to be sick. You have too much to do. Just tell that old dust storm it's not going to mess with you tonight. No way are you getting sick." Pretty soon she was breathing up a storm—that thought made her laugh: breathing up a storm.

Right away Carol started to relax. "I could feel my bronchial tubes and lungs opening up. I could see it clearly, by visualizing. The lungs were like wings spreading themselves to fly, loaded with life-giving oxygen.

Carol had to learn patience, to slow down when the signals started mounting in her head. People have different weaknesses—with some it's the stomach, with others, headaches and backaches. With Carol it's her breathing. When her breathing starts giving her trouble, she gives the rest of her body permission to relax and rest.

Carol is big on goals, and she motivates herself. "Like Gladys said, you have to have a goal bigger than yourself. This gets you away from being preoccupied with every little thing wrong with you. I think of my writing as one of those goals. If they didn't pay me to do it I'd still be interested in getting around and talking to people. It's fun sometimes to see how different people can be. There are some, about whom you never hear, who have a nobility about them, who give to others in a quiet and caring way. Others skim the surface of life lightly—politicians are often like this—when they should be delving into things and thinking what they could be doing for people.

"Gladys was more of a partner than a mentor. She'd say, 'If you have a hunch about something, something that's just not going right, listen to that hunch. The hunch came out of some-where, your subconscious mind, your physician within, and simmered to the top of your head.' She'll tell you what to try, a new exercise like tai chi, or an allergy pill with no side effects. She never says, 'I'm going to cure you.' She says, 'It's the God in you, the master physician that heals.'

"From listening to Gladys, I've learned when to ease off. Like she says, 'Your body tells you.' You learn to meditate some, to mingle with nature, to enjoy the flowers in the spring, to sit in the warm glow of the sunshine, to take a meal with a friend. Gladys walks her talk. She does the same thing in her own life that she tells her patients to do. She meditates. She eats her veg-gies and fruits, tosses in a little red meat on occasion. She exer-cises and gets massages. Here she is in her 70s, when most people are declining, and she's traveling around to Europe, India, China. People half her age couldn't handle her schedule. She's got a great goal driving her on—wanting to help people. You can't beat that one.

"Gladys also got me thinking about my everyday life. That's where the real crunch comes. You have to get the negativity out of your life. It's a killer. And you have to eliminate negative people from your life, the vexatious ones. A lot of women have parents and spouses and bosses telling them they can't do this and they can't do that. I'm a very independent type. Fighting for your life since you were a kid does that for you. I told my hus-band when we married—he was a newspaper reporter as well—'I'm going to do whatever I please as long as it's within reason, doesn't break any laws, and doesn't hurt anyone else.'"

Carol is constantly challenging herself. Challenges are often the spice of life, but you can't go beyond your normal parameters and strength. Once Carol hurt herself while riding a balky horse bareback in her spacious backyard that served as a corral.

The first person she called was me. And I, her physician who knew her so well, could hardly believe it. She didn't look big enough or strong enough to mount a horse, and this was a strange horse to begin with, one she had been boarding and had never ridden. Now she had tried to ride him without a saddle. The horse wasn't schooled, and he balked at a strange rider, taking off at a gallop, bucking like a bronco, heading for a fence with barbed wire running across the top of it. Carol kept cool, realizing that if the horse ran her into the barbed wire it could be a disaster. She decided to bail out as the fence got uncomfortably close, picking her spot to fall, one where she could land and not be run over by the horse. She hit the ground like cement. The horse was coming back after her, but she managed to roll over, and her son then waved off the horse.

Carol knew she had broken something. We later found out that it was her pelvis and tailbone. Lying there in pain, she thought of her two natural birth experiences, when she diverted the pain with music and with visualizing the opening of a lotus flower and the flowing of a waterfall. Now, when they brought her into the house, she asked her son to play some soothing music for her.

Her husband chided her for mounting the horse without a saddle. Carol said she had been instructing him. "Stop instructing him," her husband said. "He doesn't speak your language."

It could have been a tragedy, but Carol made a learning experience of it. She lay flat on her back for three months, listening to some relaxing music tapes I had given her. Meanwhile, she was also cooking up ideas for new projects.

"Everything happens for a reason," I told her. "If you don't learn certain lessons the easy way, you learn them the hard way."

Twenty-four hours before the accident, Carol had been flying back from New York where she had attended a writers' conference. Sitting in the plane thinking of all the things she had to do, all the bustling around, all the deadlines, she told herself, "I wish I could find a way out of this merry-go-round."

And she found it. On a horse.

"When you have this inner connection," I told her, "you have to be careful what you ask for. You may get it."

Mercury's Insidious Impact

*We took the fillings out.
The chest pain went away.*

—Dr. Cecil Barton

They came with aches and pains that had no name. There was a numbness of the hands and feet, a twinge in the joints, dizziness and headaches, and a strange malaise that made it an effort to turn over in bed. Some had symptoms of multiple sclerosis (MS), a lack of equilibrium and coordination. Yet they tested negative for MS and any other disease.

As I thought more about it, I realized I had tested every part of these particular patients' anatomies but their gums and teeth. These symptoms were so diverse it hardly seemed likely they came from the same source. Yet toothaches often reflect secondary infections elsewhere in the body.

I started sending some of these patients to a dentist who practiced holistic medicine and who checked the health history of every patient who came to him for a problem connected with the teeth.

Dr. Cecil Barton served on the board of the non-profit educational research foundation that bears my name. He was thorough and open, the only dentist I knew who sat his patients down and had a talk with them about their personal problems. I was impressed. Soon reports began drifting back. Dr. Barton had noted a link between body disorders and those shiny white, evenly spaced grinders in the patient's mouth. The teeth weren't the culprits, but the base metal fillings, the alloys of silver-mercury and crowns of nickel-chrome, were. He removed scores of these fillings, and in many cases the health problem was quickly removed. The reason was obvious: mercury, and its insidious impact, slowly infiltrating the human system.

We discussed the situation to some extent. From down-to-earth practical experience with patients, Barton had established that mercury has a habit of seeping out of silver fillings as vapor, abraded particles and corrosive products. These are inhaled or ingested directly by tissues. Temperature and a zinc plating influence vaporization, and the abrasion caused by chewing increases vaporization.

As Barton explained, in addition to the vapor inhaled and the particles swallowed, there's a local activity whereby mercury migrates directly into the adjacent tissues—the gums, tooth structures and jawbone—and may then spread through the system.

"Changes over the years in the metals put in the mouth," said Barton, "have some bearing on the increasing mercury menace. Traditionally, caps and inlays were made out of gold alloys, covered with plastic or porcelain. When the price of gold went sky-high, some dentists began using cheaper metals. These metals were harder, but they shouldn't have been put in anyone's mouth. Any metal put in the mouth in the presence of saliva—an electrolyte capable of conducting an electric current—becomes a battery and starts generating currents or negative charges. Precious metals like gold and platinum give off a positive charge. The negative charge metals often affect the nervous system. Some people get a shock from them.

"With silver-mercury fillings," he stressed, "grains of mercury trickle out every time someone eats hot food, or chews down on food, creating friction. The American Dental Association says, 'Yes, some mercury comes out, but not enough to worry about.' Not for who to worry about?"

Barton's explanation clarified many ailments I couldn't otherwise have accounted for, and there lies the value of keeping an open mind. A Duke University product, Barton's credentials are impeccable. He's been a holistic dentist for 30 years, treating people and not just their teeth. His primary interest is in patients, his and other physicians', who have been unnecessarily exposed to health hazards when seeking health care.

"There is no safe amount of mercury," Barton says. "Mercury is a poison. We've shown through animal studies with sheep and monkeys that the mercury from dental fillings impairs kidney functions and suppresses the immune system, and may be a culprit in additional disorders.

Barton laid it all out in what I considered a scientific manner. It worked. What could be more scientific? Perhaps the best test of all was the disappearance of so many different illnesses after the mercury fillings were removed. The Swedish government has banned these fillings for pregnant women. Others make the dentist inform the patient when using mercury which can potentially cause birth defects. Barton saw progress.

"A correlation between a tooth infection and an aching shoulder or arm has been generally accepted. The infected tooth is extracted and the infection is cleared—the same nervous system is involved. I once had a patient in his 40s, with a chronic intermittent pain in his chest. He kept choking for air, and his doctors had him on aspirin and blood thinners for years. He also had six silver mercury fillings, one in a wisdom tooth. When we took the fillings out, the chest pain went away. It never came back. His case was not unusual, but the medical establishment calls them "anecdotal experiences." It won't accept them as fact unless you put the filling back in a patient's mouth and the pain repeats itself. This is 'controlled repetition,' and that's scientific, the establishment says. But the body and mind don't care about that. They function their own way."

Just as mercury, also used in the manufacture of hats, had a harmful effect on the so-called "Madhatters," it may also have had some effect on dentists, who have been tabbed with a high suicide rate. Barton has seen a good deal of mercury-related stress and depression. "It's a mistake to take mercury poisoning lightly. Mercury is 50 percent of a silver filling. Silver, copper, tin and zinc make up the rest. When the mercury's mixed, there may be vaporizations for various reasons. The people who mix this composite are exposed to it. Nobody is immune.

"Mercury's a ravager. It can cause abdominal problems, killing helpful bacteria in the digestive tract, creating candida and yeast disorders. Mercury combines with food to create desserts the yeast love to feast on. They thrive on it—and the human system. Mercury is a neurological menace, affecting the nervous system and everything connected to it—insomnia, depression, emotional instability, memory loss, headaches, tremors, numbness and tingling in the limbs, convulsions, epilepsy, lupus, Parkinson's disease."

And this is only a partial list.

Barton's an unusual dentist, a pioneer in treating the whole person, not just a tooth. "I first meet a patient outside the dental environment," he says. "We discuss their past experiences. I try to get some idea of their values, stress level, domestic life and their fears—particularly where dentistry's concerned. We work together at relaxing and erasing those fears. So often a mother will say to a child about the drilling, 'Don't think about it. It only hurts for a little while.' The word 'hurt' may stay with them for a lifetime. We get them de-stressed instead of distressed—with no grinding of teeth and clenching of jaws, which only add to the tension and abrasion."

Like myself, Barton believes the weakest part of the anatomy should be strengthened to maintain the health of the whole. That weakness all too often is something related to the mouth: teeth, gums, tongue, cheek insides, fillings.

"I let the patient know I'm there to help in any way I can. The patient can talk to me about anything, giving the physician within free rein. I can spout all I want, but no one cares how much you know until they know you care. They listen as I give them a choice of fillings and crowns. I don't do mercury and I tell them why. They can have gold alloy, which is more expensive, or quartz covered by plastic or porcelain. Quartz is safe. You don't have to debate it. I want health-conscious patients to take charge of their bodies and anything else that affects their general health and the teeth. The two are indivisible.

"Many dentists have become tooth carpenters. They look at a tooth. They see a structural or a dollar challenge. We look at the patient. All of the patient. We want patients to educate themselves on the importance of nutrition and exercise for bone structure. Teeth are held in by the bone. Trace minerals like manganese, potassium, calcium and magnesium are important in bone metabolism and teeth metabolism. Patients can get the calcium in raw milk or yogurt, the potassium in oranges, bananas and potatoes. Or they can take vitamin supplements.

"I want patients to know what we're dealing with. It's not just brushing and flossing your teeth. The place where your teeth are housed has a lot to do with keeping the same teeth for the rest of your life. How strong is the body? The immune system? Bone structure is vital. If the bone goes bad, the teeth get loose, and that's periodontal or gum disease. The outer portion of the tooth is inert, inorganic, probably like ivory. Underneath is a living substance that is like bone. Inside this are blood vessels and nerves. So the teeth have life. The outside may be harder than bone, but teeth are not resilient. Patients soon see that the blood vessels and nerves in their teeth connect to the rest of their body. If their body is mercury sensitive, or nickel sensitive, they'll soon know about it.

"I have patients with some insight into their illness. Something they gleaned for themselves, or with Gladys. Like this patient with the chest problem. He actually figured it out for himself. But if he'd gone to the average dentist and asked to have his silver fillings removed, they would probably have thought he was crazy. I listened to him. I knew enough of what the mercury did to do what he wanted. And what the situation called for. We were simpatico. Each wanting what was best for him. And the therapist, me, listening to the patient's physician within."

Fear—the bugaboo in dental care as well as in broader health care—is always the enemy. Barton works against fear. "About 50 percent of the population seeks dental care on a crisis basis and that so often compounds the fear. It's so much easier to handle a dental problem before it reaches a climax of infection and pain. You need to eliminate the fear that keeps a child—or a grown-up—out of the dentist's chair, but you need to be careful about how you do it. For example, a parent who 'assures' a child with words like, 'He uses a long needle that he sticks in your mouth to put the tooth to sleep. But it won't hurt you,' may be doing more harm than good."

Barton smiled. "Now who would believe that one? Surely, no self-respecting six-year-old boy. But for the properly forewarned six-year-old, there is no pain. The anesthetizing procedure is over before he knows it. Those who have become comfortable with their dentists look forward to their appointments. They understand that they're doing something for themselves."

I have followed Barton closely over the years. A dozen years ago, when he began replacing mercury fillings, many Arizona dentists looked on him as a quack—or worse. They said he was doing this just to make money. But Barton saw immediate changes in the health of children and adults, and that kept him going. His patients helped too. They talked about how their other health problems had been alleviated and that quieted some of the criticism.

There were mercury horror stories. Barton talked about a child, seven-year-old Teresa, who had something called Milk Bottle Syndrome. "Sometimes, when mothers make a habit of putting children to bed with a bottle of juice or milk, there's a lot of tooth decay and the baby teeth literally rot. Teresa went through county dental care. In the office of the county pedodontist, a children's dentist, they did what they normally do in such a case. They tied Teresa on a board, sedated her, put chrome crowns on nearly all her teeth and put a large silver-mercury filling in one tooth. When she smiled, you saw all these chrome teeth."

A neurological problem developed with the fillings. The child began limping, and her arm would drag. Her face sagged and she drooled out of the corner of her mouth. She had mental lapses and became cranky. Before this, she was a model child.

The mother must have listened to the physician within because she had a strong feeling that these conditions were related to the fillings, even though the doctors had told her that Teresa had a rare genetic disease affecting her nervous system.

The mother trusted her physician within and brought the child to Dr. Barton. The crowns appeared to be nickel-chrome, and many people are allergic to nickel. The mother wanted the caps removed and the child was agreeable—she didn't like her chrome smile. Dr. Barton did two or three teeth at a time, 12 in all. The change was amazing. The child's health improved almost immediately and the neurological symptoms vanished. Nothing else but the dental work was done, and the child had received no new medications. Yet she was a totally different person, attentive, friendly and able to concentrate. She moved around easily, walking without any sign of a limp. She slept better and had more energy. She went back to school, no longer listless or tired. The case history says it all.

Age was no consideration. He removed the silver fillings of a middle-aged couple with aches and pains. They were impressed by the result. Their teenage son was having emotional problems—all he did was sit around the house, drinking Cokes, smoking cigarettes, listening to rock music. They made an appointment for him. On the routine questionnaire requesting his occupation, he wrote, "mental patient."

"He had nine silver-mercury fillings," Barton recalls. "We removed all of them in one session, replacing them with a harmless plastic. Within two or three days he turned his life around. He found a job, stopped smoking, changed his diet, and took an interest in improving his life. His parents were amazed and delighted. Their lives changed as well."

Obviously, the mercury had an impact on the immune system. Not in all people, but in enough to make it a major problem. More and more people were becoming aware of the menace lurking in their mouths. One of Barton's aides thought her sister might be helped. She had a severe case of acne, embarrassing at times for a pretty girl. Bonita got her mercury fillings removed. Within six weeks her face cleared up, and it's been clear ever since.

When there is disharmony in the mouth, with conflicting electric currents, there may also be disharmony in the mind and body. A woman had gone to a homeopathic physician with a burning sensation on her tongue and on the floor of her mouth. It kept her from sleeping. She mentioned that she'd just had a cap put on a tooth on the left side of her jaw. The physician knew something about the mercury problem and he referred her to Barton.

Barton discovered a variety of metals in this woman's teeth. "The new crown was nickel-chrome. We could tell by the electrical charge. There was also a gold crown. The dissimilar metals, with contrasting electrical currents, were causing the irritation. We took off the nickel-chrome crown and the pain disappeared. We made her a new gold and porcelain crown and that ended her problem."

Some dentists and physicians accused Barton of practicing witchcraft, but it didn't bother him. "It's the kind of witchcraft we should have more of," he said. "For the patient's sake. That's what we're all about—helping people." Barton recalled working with an older woman who had a numbness in her legs and arms. "We were removing the fillings from her lower right jaw when she suddenly raised her hands and started rubbing them together. She was crying so hard that tears were flowing into her mouth. I stopped working and asked her what was wrong. She continued to cry as she said, 'The feeling is coming back to my fingers. I haven't felt those fingers in seven years, and now the feeling is coming back.'

"The feeling came back as we were removing the fillings," Barton said. "This was one of those days when I couldn't care less what some of these dentists were saying about me."

Other dentists have been doing similar work and trusting their own experiences. Dr. Tom Hirsch in Malibu, California is one of them. "I haven't put mercury fillings in a patient's teeth for years," Hirsch told me. "And I've taken them out of 500 mouths.

I do these removals regularly. Only the other day I had a woman with a scaly rash all over her hands. I took out her silver fillings and replaced them with a quartz composite. In a week or two the rash was gone. It's amazing the way it works."

A new patient once walked into Hirsch's office. He was down in the mouth, shoulders sagging and looking beat up. "I didn't ask him what was bothering him. I didn't want to get into anything that might pull him down even more. He was slumped in the chair, not saying anything. I was probing at an old bridge and I nicked out a piece of silver. He immediately sat up in the chair. 'I don't know what you did,' he said, 'but I feel a release, like I'm a new person. I feel alive.'"

Hirsch believed that the mercury from the filling was getting into the patient's nervous system, affecting his energy in some way. He removed the old bridge and replaced it with a new mercury-free bridge. "It turned the man's life around," Hirsch recalled. "Almost immediately he became calm and composed. With a new positive energy."

Many of Hirsch's mercury patients were walk-ins. The physician within was telling them that their problems could be related to their teeth, even though their teeth weren't hurting. Other patients were referrals from Theresa Dale, a certified naturopathic physician—not an M.D.—who had become interested in teeth analysis while studying magnetic field therapy and homeopathy in Germany.

Like Hirsch, Dale practiced in Malibu. Her attitude is cautious. "There's no sure prognosis. With some patients the relief is immediate. For others it may take months before the mercury is detoxed from their system. It depends on the individual. I have seen some multiple sclerosis patients helped immediately with the removal of mercury fillings, but it may take months with other patients. Emotional people are more sensitive to mercury and react quicker. Mercury also burdens the immune system.

Some people don't have a problem with it at all, because of their stolid nature and a stable environment. In big city areas where there is more stress, mercury appears to affect people more frequently. I also always test people to see if it would be best to treat them with porcelain or gold. You don't want to replace the mercury with another toxic substance.

"No parent should allow a dentist to put mercury in a child's teeth, to start them off in life with toxic metal in their mouths. It doesn't matter if the mercury's covered with porcelain. It seeps through. A tooth is an organ and it's porous."

It may take years for mercury's effects to manifest themselves. In the meantime, it quietly works its way through the human system, lowering its immunity and leaving the individual fatigued or otherwise indisposed. Then, as it did with one woman, it may erupt painfully into an ugly and frightening welt.

Thirty years after an automobile accident in which she suffered a broken jaw, Lois Gibson, the wife of comedian Henry Gibson, noticed a mole-like growth on her jaw. She didn't connect it with the accident, which occurred a lifetime ago, and neither did her doctors. A dermatologist, with a long face, told her it looked like something that might become cancerous.

Frightened half out of her wits, she lost no time consulting a Los Angeles plastic surgeon, Dr. Cadvan Griffiths. He shook his head and diagnosed it as an incipient infection, nonmalignant, and ordered immediate X-rays, suspecting that the infection had gotten into the jawbone. In subsequent surgery, Griffiths cut into the bone and found what appeared to be a pea-size nugget of mercury in the soft tissue next to the bone. It had apparently been driven there by the accident years before. There were also scattered granules of mercury throughout this area, so small they could hardly be seen. He extracted these as well.

"The mercury had been progressing through her body for

some 30 years. Fortunately, it finally expressed itself on the skin's surface. The surgery cut down appreciably on the mercury her body had to deal with, and it eased the physical and emotional stress she was undergoing."

Lois Gibson felt an immediate rise in her energy and spirits. "Amazing," she said, "that all this could be going on in my body without my knowing about it."

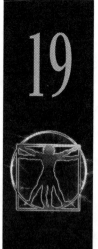

Of Fear and Pain

Much of your pain is self chosen.
It is the bitter potion by which
The physician within you
Heals your sick self.

—Kahlil Gibran

"Yes," I often repeat to my patients. "Yes, pain may be good for you. It tells you where you're hurting, and it tells you how sick you are. It's a form of social communication. If you have a pain in the shoulder, one of the things you might ask is, 'Am I shouldering too much?' If you have a pain in the neck, the question may be twofold: 'What is it I'm being a pain in the neck about?' Or, 'Who am I allowing to give me a pain in the neck?'"

I have thought about pain often, supervising so many births, treating so many cancers, holding so many hands when nothing more could be done.

Many of us think that having a healthy abundant life means we should have a life free of pain, but that doesn't necessarily follow. Pain isn't the real adversary. In reality it's not pain we're dealing with, but fear. Gripped by fear we do everything we can to control or moderate our pain and we become addicted in the process. What are the most common medications? Pain-killers and tranquilizers. We want to keep the pain out there, away from us. We think that as long as we don't deal with it, it will go away. What we have to do is work with the pain, flow with it and know that at times it is necessary.

I knew a patient, 25 years old, with a low back pain so severe that every step was excruciating. Doctors had recommended surgery to numb the affected nerves, but the physician within led the patient—by what appeared to be chance at the time—to a chiropractor I respected. He took one look at the young man crawling into his office and stretched him out on a massage table. He measured his legs and said, "Together, one leg is two inches shorter. Individually, they're the same length. You're out of joint."

With one thrust he put a displaced sacroiliac joint back in place. The relief was instant. Had the nerves been deadened, the patient might never have known the blessing of a warning pain. He empathized with women, like his wife, who dreaded the wrenching pain of bearing a child.

I told him it didn't have to be that way, particularly in nat-ural birthing where we show the young mother how to get involved with pain and plug into it. Some plug out. I was deliv-ering a child at home, and the mother belonged to some reli-gious group who did a lot of chanting to get their energy level up to where they could commune with the Great White Father. She also knew something about meditation. She decided that when she went into labor she was going to separate herself from the contractional pains she'd heard about from every young mother she knew.

During labor she was in quite a bit of pain, and the meditation wasn't working. She turned to an aide she was comfortable with and said, "This hurts."

The aide assisting me noted that nothing was happening. The muscles weren't contracting and the baby was staying in there. The mother was doing nothing to help. She had detached herself from the birthing process but not from the pain. The aide patted her on the tummy. "I know it hurts," she said. "Now let's get on with it."

The cervix was dilated one centimeter, a fraction of an inch. The mother was groaning, lying on the bed without moving her body. I had told her she should ride out the pain. Because we knew something about her chanting, the aide suggested a chant that they could do together. She said, "Dear, we are going to start chanting: 'Open lotus, open lotus.'" And as nice as you please, the lotus opened—to a full 10 centimeters. Now it was time for her to start pushing, but she couldn't push.

The aide said, "Dear, it's just like having a bowel movement," but her baby was hardly a bowel movement and there was no way she was going to do that. The next suggestion was to chant, "Down and out. Down and out." For a half-hour or so they chanted: "down and out" until the baby was down and out. The mother delivered this baby nicely, and was so busy chanting that the pain didn't stop her.

In another home delivery, I decided to use acupuncture to ease the mother's pain during the delivery of her second child. The mother had expressed the fear that the baby, exceptionally large, might rupture the vaginal membranes too soon in its determination to get born. The pain which came with the contractions was inevitable.

The acupuncture seemed to help. The mother relaxed and the dilation took place. Everything was fine and homey. The child I had delivered two years before was an interested observer, fascinated by the shiny medical instruments. The mother had remained quiet, not so much as a groan, until the point at which the baby was born. It was 11 pounds and the mother let out a blast that could have been heard a block away. Her two-year-old got so scared that he ran out of the room. Finally, his curiosity got the best of him and he edged into the doorway, wanting to see what was going on. I didn't want him to relate the birth of his little brother with fear or pain, so I called to him and said, "Now, Bobby, did you hear the loud, happy noise that your Mommy made when your baby brother was born?" He looked at me and his eyes widened. "Loud, happy noise?" he repeated. I said, "Yes, loud, happy noise." So we talked a little bit about loud, happy noises. Later, his father said that that was all the child talked about. He had backed off at an indication of pain, just as his elders so often did, but once he associated it with a happy event, he was fine, singing "happy, happy noise." The whole family rejoiced with him.

Some ask: Which came first? Fear or pain? It really doesn't matter. They are joined and live in the same house.

We had this young man with a kidney problem. He was 21, but his kidneys had stopped growing when he was 14. He was already on the dialysis machine when he came to us and he hated every moment of it. He found it degrading that he needed anything like this to keep his urine flowing. He'd been on dialysis for three or four years, and thought of it as his nemesis. We worked with diet and with the castor oil packs placed over the kidney area, but we didn't make any appreciable progress. Then we went on to his visualizing himself to health: seeing his kidneys as a pair of leathery pumps, sending the water flowing into a bladder that looked like a football. He liked that. His dislike of the dialysis machine, however, was so personal that we felt he had to overcome this aversion before he could really start getting anywhere. We had him work with his dreams, both to get his subconscious mind moving and to look for any message of hope they might contain. Mainly, we worked on trying to get him to like the dialysis machine and to see it as a friend rather than an enemy.

The clue to his struggle came one day when he exploded angrily after a session with the dialysis: "That damn thing keeps me from doing everything I want to do."

That was all I needed. I saw this anger as his physician within, striking out at a machine that had come to symbolize his weakness as a human being.

"Why," I said, "don't you see it as a friend? Visualize it as your helper. Let it heal you instead of hurting you. Make it real personal. Give it a name. Think of it, when you visualize, as a guy who's keeping you alive, so you can do more of the things you're doing. Draw a picture of what he looks like to you. He's your friend. Your special friend."

I saw a smile break out over his face. The idea appealed to him. Then came a frown. "Suppose I don't see anything?"

"You can't think that way, not when you visualize. You don't want your conscious mind to get into that. Just tell yourself it's going to work. Know that the healing process starts with you, and your friend—whatever you call him."

One week later he came flying into our clinic, running all the way. "I peed this morning. I peed. Charlie did it."

"Charlie," I frowned. "Who's Charlie?"

"Charlie, my dialysis machine. My friend, Charlie. Don't you remember?"

I remembered. It had worked.

Fear and pain are so closely bound they might as well be twins. Fear and pain had immobilized the arm of a young woman who came to our clinic. She carried her arm on a pillow when she walked in. She couldn't lift it. Nobody could even hug her, our usual welcome for the sick and fragile. She was hurting and made no secret about it. That was fine. She didn't try to detach herself from her pain. We taught her about visualization, and she would visualize herself throwing a baseball and let her subconscious mind roll with the pain. It's a lot easier to heal something physical with the inner mind because the brain sends the healing message directly to the infirmity, just as it does with a cut or a bruise. There's no chance of a short circuit. I also suggested that she send a message to her third chakra, which is the adrenal gland, where fear sits in judgment. The healing energy has to move beyond this third chakra to the fourth chakra, which deals with love. When this energy moves into the love chakra, we know what Jesus meant when he said that perfect love cancels out all fear. This is what occurs when you believe in yourself and the physician within.

Even without pain there is often an awareness that can be a blessing. While visiting in the East, I ran into a friend, an airline pilot who I hadn't seen for some time. He looked particularly fit. He had lost weight, his color had improved and he looked years younger.

"You've slimmed down," I said.

He smiled. "I lost 40 pounds."

He had had a pain in his chest, nothing serious but it could have been had it gone unchecked. It was a heart spasm. The extra poundage throughout his body, inside and out, put a strain on the circulatory system. With exercise and diet he put the problem away. He was in the best shape he'd been in for 20 years, thanks to a blessing in disguise: a pain with a message.

One of my elderly ladies had a problem with her teeth and gums but hadn't sought medical help. She was insensitive to pain in this area because of nerve damage. The infection spread through her mouth. The gums and teeth were rotting away and she didn't know it. Extensive and painful surgery was now called for. A year or so earlier it would have been an office call.

Another patient of mine, a middle-aged woman, had done well with her cancer of the colon. She had fought fear and pain with equal determination, bent on smothering her fear. Just the thought of having cancer was almost enough to have given it to her if she hadn't had it. The word terrified her. She wanted to put it behind her, along with any memory of it. She improved with diet, with exercise and with visualizing the cancer being washed away by a flow of lava, which in her mind had an irresistible effect on everything it moved against. Cancer was not normally something a right-thinking person tinkered with. You took on the pain and the fear, and looked this monster in the eye until one of you walked off the mat a winner. And she felt she had it beat.

She decided to end the therapy and get rid of even the thought of cancer. She was feeling as well as she ever had. It was time to disown the cancer and go on with the new burst of energy her inner voice had given her. I thought she was a little premature for safety's sake, but the decision was the patient's. It had been a kind of mystical experience between us, our two minds zooming in together on a common cause. Now on her own, she felt some uneasiness every now and then, having dropped everything as she had. She had been dreaming nightly in her new get-well approach, and though *she* had left the healing process, the healing process hadn't left her. When I get my patients dreaming, I know then that they are working out of the physician within. Who is a better custodian of a dream than the dreamer?

She kept dreaming after treatment, and kept a pencil and pad on her night table to remind her of the dream when she woke up. One dream, which she jotted down the moment she got up, was very vivid and in color, in deep shades of blue. Blue, as she knew, is a color symbol for truth and integrity. The dream immediately caught her attention.

She had dreamt that she and her daughter were traveling on a train in Europe with friends. They were on the way to the City of New Life. The train stopped and they got off. They were in the station when she realized in her dream that she had got off too soon. She could tell from the signs that they had not reached their destination, the City of New Life, and she had to get back on the train.

Her dream told her that she was avoiding what had to be finished, and that she was trying to deal with the cancer by not thinking about it. In the dream she saw she had to get her life in order, send her daughter off to school and check out the cancer.

She had dropped her therapy in real life, moving ahead of my timetable. The thought of having cancer had been a blight on her mind. In removing this blight she believed she'd be banishing a cancer that already showed signs of leaving. The dream told her she wasn't ready for the new cancer-free life—not yet. She'd have to climb back on the train, finish her therapy and conquer the fear that even the thought of cancer invoked.

Fear had brought her to the wrong decision at first. The physician within, the dream, pointed out her mistake. She went back to therapy, and finished what she had to do. It all worked out.

I was told in medical school to never give people false hope. Through the years I have come to believe that there is no such thing as false hope. Hope is a spiritual quality, something a patient can always build on. You can give false expectations, and that is entirely different. A doctor should never tell a patient that he or she is going to get well when that doctor's perception is different. On the other hand, if a doctor says, "You've got cancer and six months to live," it may be like signing a patient's death warrant. Whether a person consciously thinks about it or not, the body, with its innate intelligence, says: "I've got six months to live."

On the other hand, if the physician, in all honesty, can give the patient even the slimmest ray of hope, the patient may latch onto this. Whether consciously visualized or not, the body understands and thrives on that sprig of hope. Many patients who didn't appear to have the slightest chance of recovery have nevertheless risen up like a phoenix out of the ashes, fully recovered.

As friends and relatives die off, many people find themselves facing the lonely years with fear and a feeling of emptiness. As they roll back the years, they often wonder what their lives were all about, or they think of how little they have accomplished outside of their family, which is no longer in place. These are hardly the Golden Years we've heard about, but they can be good years when we have a goal, however small, and the belief that there is somebody who wants us to stay around a while and enjoy the universe he created.

A woman came to me, hopelessly depressed. She was in her 70s. It was an effort, physically and mentally, to rouse herself out of bed in the morning. After she poured her morning coffee and had a bite of cold cereal, there was nothing for her to do. She could have gone for a walk, read the newspaper, gone down to the library or offered herself for voluntary work. But none of these things occurred to her.

She was immersed in her own loneliness and pain, and it never went away. And she perpetuated it with her downbeat attitude. She had finally come to me because she had heard through the grapevine that I sat my patients down, talked to them and encouraged them to talk to me. It took time, but what better can a doctor do with her time?

The woman had come to Arizona from another state, hoping

to find a friendlier environment in a place where the sun always shone and people walked around in their shirtsleeves. She hadn't found the friendliness she was seeking because she was diffident and held back from people out of fear. She would have loved it if another person, another woman, had walked up to her and asked who she was and where she came from, but nobody was about to do that, not when she went about with a face that was frozen by years of loneliness and pain.

She came in to the clinic a few times. There was nothing radically wrong with her physically. She had a little of what she called rheumatism—and now arthritis—and a raspy throat at times from the dry desert air, but on the whole she had a sound body and a mind craving attention. By getting her to meditate on scenes from childhood that meant something to her—a red rose, a dying sun in shimmering gold, the violets in a garden she once cultivated—we opened her visual mind little by little, preparing her for a subconscious experience, for dreaming. I told her to keep a dream book on the table beside her when she went to bed.

The woman smiled deprecatingly. She had been this way for several years, deprecating of herself. It had come with a solitary, empty life. "I never dream," she said.

"Yes you do," I said, "we all dream. We just don't remember our dreams unless we tell ourselves at bedtime that we will dream and remember."

For a moment a bemused look came over the woman's face. "That sounds delightful. My own little movie at home."

I had never thought of it that way, but her comment brought a smile to my face.

"I am sure more than ever that you will have a lovely dream."

A few days later the woman brought in her dream. It was so on the mark that it raised my eyebrows. In this dream she saw milk bottles on her front porch like in the good old days when the milkman delivered milk and stopped by once a week to collect his money. Two of the bottles were labeled Doubt and Fear. Two others bore the labels Faith and Trust.

I wanted to hug the woman and squeeze her close, but this was a time to be analytic and judicious.

"And which did you choose?"

The woman smiled and her face seemed 20 years younger.

"I got the message. I got rid of my Doubt and Fear, thanks to you."

"No," I said, "you did it. It was that inner connection we talked about—the physician within you."

The dream was more explicit than a road map. In her dream, the woman picked up the Faith and Trust bottles and brought them into her house. She left the Doubt and Fear bottles on the doorstep. This dream was a major turning point for her. She began to consciously work on the faith and trust aspects of living and she found her life expanding. She made many friends, joined a church group and did some volunteer work.

I didn't see her for some time. There was no reason to because she had found what she needed through the physician within (and a little nudge from the physician without).

I have also found the biofeedback machine useful in coping with pain, once patients become aware of their subconscious powers. A young athletic-looking woman had come into the clinic with an aching shoulder that was driving her up the wall. I checked her over, then sent her to Fred Wechsler, a clinical psychologist. She had been to orthopedic doctors, rehab specialists and neurologists. They couldn't find anything with X rays, which don't spot injuries to the soft tissue, but she was in pain virtually all the time. Her muscles would tighten up with the least stress, physical or emotional. There was nothing I could pinpoint either, but I believed her when she said she hurt. The doctors hadn't. They decided it was her imagination, and she was beginning to wonder about it herself.

Fred had had some success with relaxing sore muscles with biofeedback through the visualization process, and I had an idea he might be able to help her. He put the electrodes attached to the biofeedback machine on her aching shoulder and she experimented with different visualizations and meditations to reduce the tension in that specific muscle. She imagined the muscle becoming soft and loose, thinking of it as Jello or a puffy cloud. Then she saw it softening and loosening like a puff of cotton. She also pictured an imaginary hand gently massaging her shoulder.

She kept repeating her imagery, judging when she was in the alpha—or healing—state by the bell-like tone of the biofeedback machine. She concentrated on visualizing what evoked that tone until the tension left the muscle and the shoulder no longer ached. She had started to believe, like the other doctors, that the pain might be all in her mind. But the visualizations accomplished what all her earlier treatments weren't able to do. Her whole body relaxed. "Now that I know it's there," she told Wechsler, "I can cope with it."

I have become accustomed to the healing energy of pain. A pain in the neck, or a headache, when constant, is enough to summon the healing mind of the physician within. Pain awakens us to a problem, and when we take pain medicines and tranquilizers instead of listening to what the pain is telling us, we are denying the healing energy of our bodies and minds which rally to our help.

As a child in India, where I became very aware of lepers and leprosy, I saw even then that the problem lepers had was not pain but the lack of it. They could inadvertently burn a hand in a bonfire and not know it was burned until they smelled the burning flesh.

Physical pain is the first consciousness we have of a hurt. If we are wise, we will promptly do something about it. Consult a doctor, but don't let the pain run on, taking a pill or applying a salve every now and then to get by. Whatever is wrong will only get worse.

Some pains reach deeper into the human consciousness, like the emotional and spiritual pain of being cut off from God and love. This kind of pain reminds us that we should do something about reviving our communication with God. The story of the prodigal son in the Bible deals with a son being cut off from his father. When awakened to the reality of this separation, the pain hits him—but it also brings him back to his father.

Mental pain is one of our greatest scourges, but it doesn't have to be. We feel mental pain when we are cut off from relationships, from our family or from old memories. We don't have to die with this pain. We must live each day as if it's the first and last day of our life. We must keep our minds active and look for the healing energy within ourselves that will reconnect us with life. We need to build new pathways and spread our wings a little.

With spiritual pain we need to go to the source, to the creator. With meditation and prayer, patience and laughter, and with forgiveness—of ourselves and others—we can connect with the power within to bring us the inner peace we seek.

I have learned that by working with my patients, I reconnect with my own painful life situations. I can, to the best of my ability, model for them a level of love and caring, health and wellness.

A Clear Channel
to the Creator

*Hope springs
eternal in the breast . . .
Always to be blest.*

—ALEXANDER POPE

Melissa had something more than her-self to live for, and she couldn't let this thing beat her. What would her little girl do without her? She was barely five years old. Melissa was so young herself, not yet 30, but her thoughts were only for the child so dear to her, the child who looked up to her as if she could do anything. She could beat this if she tried hard enough. She kept telling herself this, all day, every day, as she worked to support herself and her child. And every night, as she put her beautiful child to sleep, she prayed

237

that she would make it through this ordeal. She spoke to God as though he were in the room.

"Please, God," she said, "for her sake, if not for mine."

It had been quite an ordeal for a single mother, but Melissa had rallied to the challenge. Conventional medicine had done everything it could. She had been radiated, but it hadn't worked. Then her good cells, as well as the bad, had been attacked by chemotherapy. Finally, they had removed her breast where the cancer had lodged. She had gone into remission, they said, but they could promise her no more than two years. All they could do was stem the predator that had invaded her body and was slowly stifling her life.

Melissa looked around for help. She would have done anything, gone anywhere. She had lost her hair to chemotherapy, and with it some of her spirit. She had lost weight and didn't look quite like the person she had been. But her hope never flagged. She couldn't afford to weaken, not even for a moment, while her little girl was with her. She was always smiling and cheerful when she and her daughter were together. She never permitted herself a tear, not until the lights had been dimmed. Then she would go into the child's room and look down at her with a sigh as she saw how peacefully she was sleeping.

Melissa began to worry as the months dragged on and tests showed that her white blood count was not as good as it had been. She couldn't sleep at night and a chill had come into her heart. She knew she needed to do something else, something more, an alternative to what she had been doing. She'd heard of biofeedback and its success in helping and succoring people. Often it helped heal them, even of cancer. She hadn't heard yet of the physician within, but enough was stirring inside her to know that she was again at risk. Had God not listened to her? Was he too busy with so many others? Or wasn't that the way it worked? She remembered someone saying that if you ask for help, he gives you strength. If you ask for courage, he gives you a challenge. It is always up to you. So be it.

Melissa came to our clinic. She had had about all the conventional therapy any one person could handle and still stay alive. Now, Dr. Wechsler, our psychologist, took charge. She was told that visualization might be helpful in keeping the cancer from recurring. Visualization was pretty much like what she had already been doing every day—meditating and praying—except now it would be geared specifically to her problem.

She was also introduced to the biofeedback machine, innocuous in itself. Wechsler let her know how painless it would be and how rewarding it could be. The biofeedback was just a control mechanism. It registered the healing alpha-theta brain waves with a soft sound of chimes that let her know that her mind had traveled from beta conscious-thinking to the infinitely more powerful and healing alpha-theta.

Once she got the hang of it, the process was easy and enjoyable. Wechsler told her in his low-key way what would happen.

"In a very brief time, with visualization, you will be able to create the alpha brain waves wherever and whenever you like—in your workplace, in the privacy of your home. Give yourself 15 or 20 minutes of daily respite, and work to keep your body free of the cancer cells while building up your natural defenses."

I monitored Melissa's progress along with Wechsler. I had explored biofeedback sufficiently to know how readily the average person could summon the alpha brain waves by visualizing. Often they would visualize the colors of the rainbow, identifying them with oranges, red apples and bananas. Or they would envision blue skies, green meadows, the purple twilight and the stars above. In this induced alpha state, patients could then tune into their own minds and bodies.

Melissa had no difficulty sounding the biofeedback chimes, then going about the job of boosting the white blood count that battled infection and strengthened the immune system.

Wechsler tried to make a game of it, getting her to relax and leave her mind open, free of the worries and concerns of the day. In the end, success depended on the patient, her physician within and Wechsler, all working together.

It was a challenge for Melissa and it gave her something to do about her own healing. Wechsler soon had her visualizing the white blood cells in her bloodstream. She saw them as little white dots. She filled the screen of her mind with them, visualizing them entering every cell of her body with their healing message. She envisioned the white cells increasing in strength, working together more efficiently. She saw them glomming onto the cancer cells, eating away at them. She pictured the cancer cells scattering, frightened and weakened, totally at bay. She imagined them dwindling, then being absorbed, oozing out of her body.

Melissa also practiced visualization at home every day for 30 or 40 minutes. She also did it at her job, on her lunch break. While relaxing in her office, she visualized the warmth of the sun in a scene in the tropics. She was able to bring on sensations of heaviness and warmth in the muscles of her arms and legs. The sun's warmth flowed into her chest and shoulders, fingers and toes. The more she visualized, the easier it was, and the more relaxed she became. The physician within was beginning to awaken, and Melissa was taking hold. It was something she liked doing, enjoying the idea of control from within and not being subject to external forces.

At Wechsler's suggestion, Melissa also visualized a swarm of ants living in a huge tree. They lived on the sap of the tree and protected the tree from invaders: termites and the like. The ants found their nourishment in the tree and their lives depended on it, just as Melissa depended on her white blood cells. She imagined the ants and the white blood cells in a similar protective mission. Whenever an alien insect—viewed as a transposed cancer cell—landed in the tree, the ants would quickly gather together and destroy the invader or drive it off.

The visualization continued with the white blood cells—the busy little ants—providing an environment for the cells to live and function in. The swarms of ants nesting in the tree, in the leaves and bark, were the infection fighters.

Melissa enjoyed this little game. She had no problem visualizing the proliferation and survival of her white blood cells exemplified by the friendly ants. And though ants were usually black, she saw them as white. "This made it easier," Wechsler noted, "for her body to get the message, since the protective blood cells are white." Melissa soon gained back the 10 pounds she lost during chemotherapy. She regained her confidence, with a consequent loss of fear.

Wechsler was pleased. "Over the course of a couple of months, Melissa's white blood count improved, as did her health. She was jubilant when she peered into a mirror, and cried, 'Look, I have my curls back.' This would have happened in any case, with the stopping of the chemotherapy, but for Melissa it indicated a healthier state of mind. Her white blood count had returned to normal."

She stopped coming in and was back working normally. This was encouraging. Yet there was always the danger of the cancer recurring, as her doctors had warned. Cancer in remission has a way of coming back. Wechsler had hoped she would continue with her visualizations wherever she was. All too often, patients with life-threatening disorders are so relieved at the first signs of recovery that they discontinue the treatment that helped them.

This happened with Melissa. She didn't come back. Two years after she went into remission, the cancer returned. She had stopped her visualizations after leaving biofeedback, while at the same time recommending the treatment to a friend with multiple sclerosis.

It was a shock when the cancer returned. Melissa had moved to a small town, bought a house and found a new job. She seemed to have everything in hand. Then, at the hairdresser's one day, while having her hair styled, she felt a crick in her neck—a sharp pain when she tried to lower her head to have her hair washed. She didn't think too much of it. But a few days later she had a cold and went to a local doctor. She mentioned the kink in her neck. He tried to loosen it, but it wouldn't budge. Knowing her medical background, he suggested she see her oncologist. With a tremor in her heart she visited the cancer specialist, and learned the cancer had come back.

She was back at square zero. A big zero. She told herself she couldn't panic, not with her daughter to think of and her own life at stake. She again received chemotherapy, the great cell killer, and got rid of the cancer in her neck area. But now it had spread from her spine to her hip, and her hair fell out again.

Her doctors were telling her to get her affairs in order and she knew what that meant. She had been through it before. But there was still a chance. There was always a chance until you gave up. Melissa was not about to give up.

A caring Fred Wechsler called. He had heard of the cancer's return, though he had not seen her since she dropped out. She was pleased to hear from him. In the background, as they talked, he could hear the happy singing and chirping of Melissa's young daughter, who approached her mother, noting with a child's concern, the glimmer of tears in her mother's eyes.

"Is it all right to be happy?" the little girl asked.

The mother held back her tears and smiled. "Yes, dear, it is good to be happy."

Melissa was disconsolate, but fighting. She felt the alpha training had helped, mentioning that she had recommended it to her friend with MS. But she had seen no reason to go on with it herself. She was better, she had thought, and so never had gone back.

Now she was back with her oncologist and ready to get on with conventional medicine's attack on the predator in her body. Melissa had known happiness. Hopefully, with God's help, she would know it again. With prayer and meditation, and a clear channel to the creator, anything was possible.

A Compassionate Healer

I listen to the patient.
I have no better source of
information.

—DR. HOWARD KELLY,
JOHNS HOPKINS MEDICAL CENTER

The poet Milton said, "They also serve who only stand and wait." At our holistic clinic in Scottsdale, they also serve who sit and listen, who comfort the patients as they take their histories, who evince their interest as they pass them on to my staff and myself, who handle themselves with patience and fortitude as they establish a rapport with people who are so often ill at ease or frightened.

"Many of them have been other routes," says Patti, the friendly first contact for patients at our clinic. "They are in pain, emotionally and physically, and we are their last resort. They've been around and they feel if Dr. Gladys can't help them, no one can. We have a lot of tough calls. We have cancer patients coming in for the first time. Just by listening to them, Gladys can usually tell what the origin of that cancer is.

"She listens as though she has all day. This makes people comfortable. She has a way of honing in and asking the questions that bring about a significant response. There is no magic. She acts like their best friend, which she is at that moment. You need to look at the patient and see pain in the eyes to know that this is the root from which everything is growing—the illness within, the suffering.

"Mostly it's women who come in or call. They call about every imaginable disease, and they call about husbands, boyfriends and fathers. They start telling you about their pain right away. They want something to start happening immediately. They don't care how much it costs or what they have to do, just that they can get in the line. They are all ages, even teenagers, because the word has spread that this is a doctor who cares and who knows. It's amazing to see the changes within patients after a few treatments.

"We had one patient, an elderly lady, who arrived in a wheelchair. We could hardly get her through the door. She was in her mid-70s. She looked so frail I didn't think she had long to go. Her color was gray and her eyes had little focus. She could barely move her hands. She looked like she had given up. She probably wouldn't have come in if it hadn't been for a friend, a longtime patient. Her husband had died a short time before and all the incentive appeared to have gone out of her life. She had become a recluse and in the process had stopped eating right and had stopped all exercise, even walking. At that age the muscles atrophy very quickly."

Patti followed the woman through the healing process. She wasn't just a case, just another patient. She was somebody to be cared for. And Patti, too, gave her a hug to let her know she was loved. Even though Patti wasn't a doctor or a nurse, she could see this was what the ailing woman lacked. It was something all too many doctors wouldn't even think about, something they weren't taught in medical school: love.

I saw the woman a few minutes later. I looked deeply into her eyes. I examined her, took tests, probed her vital signs. Then I leaned over and clasped the woman's hand. "Do you know you are a very fortunate woman?" I said. "There's hardly anything wrong with you. You've given up on life, but life hasn't given up on you. You have many good years."

I patted her on the shoulder. The touch was reassuring. "I'm putting you on a simple program of vitamin shots and regular massage. Then you can start enjoying yourself. Go for a trip or two, see your friends, go out to dinner. Take a friend or let them take you." I had inquired about the family. "Get together with your children. Let them know you want to see them. Tell them you're well, because you are well. Take an interest in your grandson. Let him bring you in here if he wants."

Tears came to the woman's eyes. The more she buried herself at home, the more unloved she thought she was. It was obvious and anyone who took the time could see that. In a few weeks the woman who looked and acted terminal was a new woman.

Patti smiles thinking about it. "She keeps us abreast of what she's doing when she comes in, sometimes with her grandson, for a vitamin booster and a massage. She goes on cruises, dines out with friends, new and old. She brings in goodies for the staff that she has baked. She's having a wonderful time. She's a perfect example of how the mind can make you sick—and get you well. She just needed to feel that someone cared enough to want her to stay around.

"Men respond in much the same vein. Gladys was what they missed in an impersonal male doctor. She is friendly and warm, yet quick and incisive in her professional judgments—and they are grateful. This one patient, a first-timer, had many problems. The most pressing was an addiction to his medications. He didn't realize he was addicted until Gladys picked up on it. She went over his behavior pattern. He saw immediately how this addiction had made a slave of him, while doing nothing for his high blood pressure and back pain, the original problems. He had gotten increasingly dependent on the drugs and was so badly addicted that Gladys recommended a rehabilitation clinic. She gave him something for the high blood pressure and he went away for several weeks. When he came in again, he was relaxed and mentioned how thankful he was that he had come to her. 'I feel badly now that I tried to get these prescription drugs from her. It was the reason I came in originally. I didn't realize I was addicted until she showed me how I was. I was coming in for the wrong reason.'

"Gladys invariably accessed the physician within in so many different disorders and patients. That was what healing was all about.

"She opens up their minds. Sometimes it takes a while, but in the end it's worth it because eventually they recognize how their emotional and mental behavior may be affecting their physical health. Newcomers call in and describe going through a trauma with a son or husband. They get into the physical symptoms: the stopped breath, the faintness, the feeling that they're about to have a stroke. She quiets them down with her own calm approach, tells them to be more aware of how their emotions and reactions affect their well-being. 'Try to keep calm. Try to relax. Go outside for a walk. Don't let things get out of hand. The one you hurt most is yourself.'

"It may not click right away, but we see with our regular patients how composed they are. They have learned the hard way. Gladys's quiet advice gives them something to think about, especially when their bodies suffer as they lose control emotionally."

Patti passes the patient on to Ernestine, a registered medical assistant (RMA) who delves deeper into the patient's history, checks their vital signs and the medical reasons for the visit. "Many of the women come in with candida, a yeast disease, which many doctors don't consider systemic. We treat it systemically with a yeast-free diet: no bread, wine, beer or cheese; some meat is okay, together with seafood and poultry; vegetables and some fruit, but no sugar or refined flour. Yeast and sugar combine to increase the problem. It manifests in the mouth, the intestinal tract and the vagina, where it may be infectious. Usually, I pick up on their condition. They come here as their last hope. They want someone to look at them as a whole person, not as a bundle of symptoms. They tell us and we listen.

"So many doctors get rid of the symptoms with medications. They treat the thrush in the mouth, the rash, the fungal skin problems, the burning in the vagina. Then it all returns, and we're back where we started, with tongues turned white and stomachs bloated.

"Vitamins and supplements balance out the new diet: vitamins A, B complex, C and E, plus garlic and acidophilus in pill form. We offer the patient a questionnaire, focusing on the candida symptoms. They look at it and say, 'I've had all this and no one can tell me what it is.' Other doctors look on each symptom as a separate disorder, but when all these symptoms disappear, patients feel as weak and tired as they did before. With our blood tests and other examinations, now we have to tell them that it's in their intestines as well."

One woman, attractive and youthful, was beside herself. She'd had candida problems for years. The symptoms would come and go like the wind on a rainy night. "I told my doctors about a chronic fatigue, a loss of sexual desire, fingernails breaking and dry scaly skin. They'd say it was all in my head, but that was about the only part of me that wasn't affected." When she was treated systemically at the Scottsdale Holistic Medical Group, the problem disappeared.

One of the massage therapists, Lynn Serrano, speaks with the clarity of youth. And she listens as she toils.

"Usually people talk about their illness or their pain as something they own. They basically have the answer to their problem. They have the answer within. So they talk, hoping to materialize that answer. It comes in dreams, in meditation, while they listen to music and while they talk around it as they're having a massage that awakens every cell in their body. They so often know they've given themselves their illness, but they're so involved in their own negativity, emotionally and mentally, that they find it difficult to break out all at once.

"There was this woman with severe arthritis, the rheumatoid type that gets in the bones. She was only about 35. She was grouchy and mean. You couldn't get a pleasant word out of her. She hurt badly, in every joint of her body. You'd say, 'Hello, are you having a good day? And she'd just grunt. She never had a smile or a thank you. She was impatient with everybody. She'd get angry when nobody came to open the door for her—even when they didn't know she was there. She used a scooter because she had trouble walking. This was all in the beginning of her visits to the clinic.

"We knew that it bothered her to move, that she was never out of pain. When she came into the clinic, she would go from an erect position to a sitting position. It wasn't like she was just sitting down. It was a massive effort. You could hear her hip bones grind, all her joints agonizing—the elbows, wrists, fingers, ankles, knees, even her jaw bones. She didn't have any cartilage in the bones, and you need cartilage for movement. Gladys still treated her holistically, as a whole person. She worked with her dreams to relax her and to get her involved in her own treatment. She worked with the pain using visualization. The woman would visualize a rose garden, a beautiful waterfall, a gorgeous sunset. She would see herself as a child romping through the meadows, happy as a lark. We could see her easing up, but she still was complaining. No matter how grouchy she was we listened, and we tried to please her. We knew where the irascibility and shortness was coming from. Even when we didn't relate it to the agony of moving an arm, a leg, a finger, we saw it in her eyes.

"She wanted to get well without surgery, holistically. She knew this was what Gladys stood for. She wanted to do it herself, with the physician within. She and Gladys talked about it. They talked about a hip replacement."

"If I have that done," she said, "I'll look on myself as a failure. It has to be something I do. I want to heal myself."

"I said to her, 'It is something you do. Only you can okay the replacement. Only you can make it heal. Only you can banish the pain. Nobody can bring you back but yourself. The decision is yours. Holistic medicine doesn't exclude conventional medicine, not when it does the job.'

"Once she felt she was in charge, her disposition improved. The replacement was made and she responded well. The rest of her was still hurting, but she would be mobile now, once she got through rehab—the rehabilitation process. Her physician within was telling her she was in command. She became gentler, began to smile occasionally. It was heartening to see the change in her. We did a lot of electroacuscope to help the cells of the body regenerate. It took time and patience on her part. Every joint in her body had to be stimulated. But now it was her healing. She owned it. We went on with the massage therapy and started some exercises.

"The change in her attitude was remarkable. 'When,' she said, 'will you be doing the other hip?'

"She was visualizing herself walking again. She saw it in her dreams, in her meditations. She was running and laughing in her subconscious, and it evolved in her conscious mind. She was taking charge.

"The surgeons replaced the other hip. She was in ecstasy during rehab. She and Gladys talked it through. Before, she had hesitated about surgery. Now she could hardly wait for new replacements: for both knees and a shoulder. She was a remarkable new patient, uncomplaining where she had always been complaining before. The new attitude came from a new head on her shoulders. She maintained her enthusiasm through the stress of three more joint replacements, five in all. She never flinched. The anger was gone. She was walking, faltering in the beginning, but gaining strength. She had a smile on her face. She never came into the clinic without giving everyone a hug, and not just because she was walking, but because someone had listened. Nobody had listened before. Modeling ourselves after Gladys, we understood her pain, her frustration, her anger. And we listened to it, to the unceasing pain, to her being so young, not yet 40, and seeing herself crippled for life.

"Dr. Gladys listened too, before surgery, during surgery and in the rehab months. The listening was paramount. The average doctor doesn't listen. They have their hand on the doorknob. The change came when she found she had a physician who cared, who wanted what she wanted, and who listened.

"The patient who couldn't walk before, walked off with a glad heart. She came back whenever she had a day off from her job, for maintenance and to visit. She takes a full body massage, keeping in touch with her refurbished limbs and joints, glorying in their strength. And she hugs every one of us. She is an inspiration to all of us, to get on with our work, helping and listening. She went on to head a support group for the handi-capped, and she had an eight-pound baby girl."

It was curious the way the physician within worked, and con-tinues to work. In listening, we helped make it happen.

Another patient, Clare, talked about losing her hearing. She didn't know how it had happened. It came about suddenly, a complete loss in one ear. She was 37, in apparently good health, and exercised and took massage. Lately, she had fallen off her health regimen, so stressed out by her job that she wasn't listening to her body. That was when she stopped hearing.

We suggested a specialist. They tested her and discovered an aneurism in her brain that had to be removed. She had brain surgery and it was successful.

"It was a blessing I lost my hearing," she would later tell us. "My body was telling my mind something. It took over, blocking out my hearing, so I would have the checkup that saved my life."

We rejoiced with her.

She had been so distracted that she hadn't been watching her dreams, and they had no message for her. She also hadn't been consciously meditating, but the subconscious, which had always been in touch with her, awakened the physician within. She didn't do anything consciously. The voice within did what it had to do to help her through. She was fine after the surgery, hear-ing well enough to converse back and forth, and grateful to an innate intelligence that had listened when she hadn't.

There were so many who needed to be heard.

Ann was the country-club type, articulate, composed, casu-ally dressed in tweeds, with a clear and open look. She was somewhere in her late 40s. Nobody would have taken her for an alcoholic. That was all behind her now, and though she tried to live for the present and the future, the past was still around, sometimes haunting her.

She felt we had similar patterns. We both had been married to doctors and we were both divorced. When I first saw her, she had come in because she was having an alcohol problem. She thought she was a social drinker, then found she couldn't get through the day without alcohol. More and more it had taken over her life, particularly after her 20-year-old son was killed in an accident by a drunk driver.

Ann went into a deep funk, asking God, as so many have, why this had to happen. Then another son was in a car accident. Her mother, whom she loved dearly, passed on. She was holding her hand when she died. After her mother's death, her father went into a massive depression—they had been married for 40-some years. The father and daughter took comfort drinking together, but it didn't help. The grief was worse afterwards.

Ann knew she had to stop drinking, had to do *something* about it. This was a path that went only one way: down. Still, she didn't think she was addicted, only drinking to excess. That's what so many alcoholics think—until they can't think anymore.

Married to a doctor, Ann had had a cure on hand whenever she had a headache or a pain. She'd take a pill or a drink. The drink was more satisfying. And two drinks were more satisfying than one, and so on. "After that first drink, it was getting so I couldn't stop. That's when I decided I'd have to do something about myself. I needed help. I was sophisticated and sensitive enough to know that I needed a counselor or a doctor who cared about me, the whole person. Having been married so long to a doctor, I thought in medical terms. I didn't want an ordinary doctor who thought of me only as an alcoholic. I wanted to be thought of as a person who used alcohol to excess, and was a composite of what she was inside and of what happened to her externally."

She was looking for a natural healer. She'd always taken this medication, or that one, whenever she was indisposed. Now she wanted to get away from all that. All it did was burden her system.

"A friend told me about Gladys. I'd heard about her, knowing she was a holistic physician who was into natural birthing and was married to a doctor. I assumed she favored natural healing."

She checked in with me and told me her story. I listened, sympathetically, to a wife divorced by a doctor. I could hardly help noting this similarity.

I saw a woman a generation younger, at loose ends after her divorce, close to her children and her father, yet drifting, not knowing what to do with her life. She had been married at 18 and had never held down a job. She was too young, too caring, to let the threads of her life get unraveled. The healing process wouldn't begin until the drinking stopped. I stressed that and she appeared to understand.

"You have to discipline yourself," I said. "And not until you manage that will the physician within you take hold and bring an end to your drinking."

This was something Ann had already surmised. She had quit many times. It reminded her of what Mark Twain had said about smoking. "It's easy to quit smoking. I've quit 100 times."

She, too, had quit 100 times.

We talked together like old friends, while the patients were stacking up in the waiting room. The years rolled back. She recalled her year in college, in nurses' training, which preceded her marriage. This stuck in my mind, and in Ann's. Something stirred inside her, subtly and slowly, with no direct earthshaking impact.

It took a while for Ann to end her drinking. The herbs and vitamins I recommended lost their effect with the alcohol. She kept on visualizing and meditating, hoping for a breakthrough. She visualized me as her physician within. It seemed to fit the mode.

"Gladys was my role model. She never lectured me, never made a judgment on my lifestyle. She was ageless. She had vitality, energy and a caring warmth that just exuded love. She was the kind of person I wanted to be. She was alone. I was living alone, and I found myself liking it. She had pulled herself together and started a life of her own after 46 years of marriage. I had my own feeling of failure and humiliation when I was divorced. I was shattered.

"As we talked together, I saw how she had pulled through and was living her life. She had a busy practice. She was all together. She wasn't a broken person. In fact, she appeared to be liberated, as though she were her own person for the first time. The thought came to me that I could be like that if I tried. I would have to do it myself. Gladys gives you a start, but you have to follow through. I looked around for something to do, some way of being useful. While I had never worked, I had briefly had that nursing training. As a nurse I'd be helping people. That's what I wanted to do, help people, like Gladys did, even if not on the same scale. I visualized what I thought I was best suited for and talked about it. Gladys listened. She always listens.

"I had decided on what I wanted: not a nurse and not a doctor. I didn't want a Ph.D. or a master's degree—a lot of paperwork. I wanted to work with people, people like myself. I wanted to counsel people with chemical and alcohol addictions. It was something I knew about and I had beaten it. With the physician within telling me all I needed was to accept the truth, I knew I could never take another drink and survive. I saw it as a deadly poison in my visualizations. I saw a bunch of drunks lying around in dark hallways, smelling of themselves. It was horrible. Life was too precious to be wasted. I went deep inside myself and meditated. I connected with my physician within. Quite often that physician was Gladys, sitting with a smile and an understanding light in her eye, saying, 'Go for it. You can do it.'"

And she did. Ann entered a community college, taking a two-year course in pursuit of a degree in counseling for chemical addiction. It brought a new lift into her life. She did some practical work in her internship, getting some insight into what it would be like. She was enthused, empathizing with the people she was working with. She had marveled at how I could jump into my day at seven every morning, and keep on until seven at night. She was 30-some years younger. I told her, "You have much to do. You are needed." Her eyes glowed. She took a deep breath. "What a wonderful feeling to be needed again," she said. I knew then I had no reason to be concerned. Ann would be filling that need.

She was in the middle of her school year when she came down with shingles. She'd had Christmas dinner with the grandkids and the littlest one had chicken pox. She got shingles, a similar virus. Shingles is no fun. She thought she was going to have to drop out of school because of the way she looked. I gave her acupuncture and an antiviral medication, and she wound up having a very light case. It only lasted two weeks or so. Then she went back to school and to her work with people.

Discounting the shingles, I was pleased at what I saw. I didn't say very much. I didn't have to. I saw a woman engaged with the world, a self-assured woman with a purpose as big as life.

I reached over and gave Ann a hug. She was very special to me. I said, "Do you remember what Jesus said about letting the dead bury the dead? Let us look ahead with hope in our heart, always looking for the rainbow after the squall."

Focus on Life

*W*hat I'm seeing is a
more uncritical acceptance of the
notion that you can think your way
out of disease. To me, it's a form
of wishful thinking.

—MARCEL ANGELL, EDITOR
New England Journal of Medicine

She was not quite 30 and she was dying. Not only was her youth slipping away, but so was her life. The cancer had spread to her chest and gone to her neck and shoulder. They called it Hodgkin's. She was a young doctor, a resident in a San Francisco hospital, and she was an embarrassment. Everything had been tried on her: full body radiation; two years of chemo. She couldn't get well and she wouldn't die. She was a fighter.

Now they said she was in remission, but she wasn't sure of this. She wasn't sure of anything. They said it might very well recur, and she couldn't handle that, not after what she'd been through. She had lost her beautiful blonde hair, but that would come back. Her skin had become dry and mottled, but that would come back, too. She had lost the capacity to have a child, and that wouldn't come back.

Her family was at wit's end about what to do next. She had been almost everywhere, to the top medical centers at Stanford, UCLA, San Francisco. A cancer specialist at the University of Chicago had even come to their California home to consult. She was in despair, but still lived with hope.

Her name was Barbara Griffiths, and there was an M.D. after it. They all called her Bonnie, because of her radiant smile and her easygoing disposition. She hadn't known whether to choose medicine or painting for a career. Many had told her she was a talented artist. But medicine was in her blood. Her father was a surgeon, and she had two brothers who were doctors.

The family was having dinner with a friend one evening when he noticed a bit of a mist in Bonnie's eyes. She smiled as he asked how she was doing. "I'm doing well," she said in a low voice, turning away so he couldn't see the tear.

The family friend had been thinking that day of an older woman he knew who had been given up as terminal by cancer specialists 20 years before. Only this morning he had spoken to her. She was very much alive, bright and cheerful, in her 70s now, and no one would have known she ever had cancer. When all else had failed, she had gone to the Scottsdale Holistic Medical Group in Arizona, headed at the time by myself and my former husband, Dr. William McGarey.

The friend turned now to Bonnie's parents, mentioning how this woman of substance and spirit had turned to the Cayce-oriented clinic as a last resort.

"I don't know how she was cured," he said. "It took some time. But this was a case where holistic medicine did what the conventional couldn't. It saved a life."

Bonnie had perked up. Her parents seemed interested.

"I could make an appointment," Bonnie said.

"Well, it's worth thinking about," her father said. "We can look into it."

His wife looked up and shrugged. "Well, nothing else has worked."

The family friend looked at Bonnie. She seemed tired, weary, drained. But for a moment her face lightened, and he saw her as he wanted to remember her: sweet and beautiful, loving life and always at the center of it, growing up with her brothers, vying with them in tennis, swimming, skiing. The young men flocked around her. She had an inner glow, and she was brainy. She went to top schools and he had a feeling she was one of the chosen few who could do whatever was in their hearts and minds. Then, out of some capricious void came the numbing pain, the dull ache, the strictures of muscles and tendons, and the dismaying diagnosis that was enough to send a tremor through the bravest heart: cancer.

After the initial shock Bonnie was able to assess her illness with the detachment of the scientist she was. The first thing, she told herself, was to keep going and not stop working or retire to her bed. One thought kept ringing in her ears: "Keep moving, keep active, keep working, keep smiling."

Many were the nights she got down on her knees and prayed in despair, asking the good Lord why this had happened to her when she was so young and just starting her own life. She looked into herself, and she looked outside herself. She had taken pleasure in helping others. Now, how could she help herself? She asked herself this over and over. She remembered every little detail of her treatment, and she recalled what her idol, Sir William Osler, an innovator of medicine at Johns Hopkins and Oxford, had once said, "You can't truly be a physician until you've been a patient."

Bonnie vividly described to me what it meant to be a patient—an experience she wanted to share with others who had suffered as she had. A radiologist herself, she was a fellow in medical education at the University of California, San Francisco Medical School, teaching medical students and researching trauma at St. Francis General Hospital. She was standing at the front of a classroom one day, talking about developing new teaching protocols and tools, observing the intent faces in her class, when her left arm suddenly began to hurt. She remembers the pain.

"At first it was a dull ache which progressed to an excruciating, constant sharp pain in both my arm and neck. I consulted an array of specialists, including orthopedists and neurosurgeons. After four months, an MRI was ordered. The machine always seemed to go down on the days of my appointments, so the diagnosis was delayed. One week before I was to present a paper to the Association of University Radiologists my neck 'exploded.' It blew up to twice its normal size on the left side, hurting beyond any human tolerance. I had heard in medical school that a kidney stone was mortal man's greatest pain. I knew better now. I ran into the chief neuroradiologist's office, begging for my MRI scan, and he ordered a chest X ray. I had had one only five months earlier and it had been read as normal. It was no longer normal. I saw the X ray and said, 'There must be some mistake. This isn't my chest.' There was this huge mediastinal mass which later on was found to be engulfing my aorta, encroaching upon the neural canal and squeezing my brachial plexus, the nerves which innervate the arm. That was the reason for the arm pain. A biopsy on my left supraclavicular (collar bone) lymph node led to the diagnosis of 'lymphocyte depleted nodular sclerosing Hodgkin's lymphoma'—Hodgkin's Disease.

"The doctors explained that this was one of the most curable cancers and if you have to have cancer, this is a good one to get. The type of lymphoma I had usually responds well to radiation therapy, but my tumor grew through the radiation treatments. After three days of radiation, I was also given emergent chemotherapy in the hospital. That was when I learned the cure can be worse than the disease: sedatives and antiemetics were mildly effective in making violent vomiting tolerable; IVs (intravenous injections) pricked, stung and then burned. My brain felt like scrambled eggs, then poached; and I was so weak that I craved vitamin B (blood transfusions).

"Very soon I became chronically anemic, and I wasn't sure if my inability to learn or to remember things was due to the 'life-saving' drugs or to my body running on half-empty. It certainly wasn't for lack of trying. Every night after my clinical rotation I would go straight home, open my books and outline the material I was studying. I tried all the tricks I learned in medical school to absorb the study material, but nothing would stick. It was as if my brain were a sieve. I wondered if I was dying and if this was part of the death process. Then I quickly tried to put the thought away. I knew that thinking of dying was no way to get well, but no one had mentioned the importance of being upbeat and cheerful, and I don't think I would have listened at this point. All the focus was on the lymphoma.

"Three months into the chemotherapy my legs went numb, and the night sweats, which I'd been having for weeks, got more frequent and longer in duration. The neurologist diagnosed radiation myelitis (inflammation of the spinal cord or bone marrow), and the gynecologist informed me that I had gone through 'premature menopause secondary to chemotherapy-induced ovarian failure.'

"I must admit I cried that night. I was 30 years old, unmarried, and they were telling me I couldn't have children. My knight in shining armor, my boyfriend and potential husband, was distraught but seemingly supportive. 'Maybe we can adopt when you get over all this,' he told me. I didn't want to adopt. I wanted to have my own. I came from a family of four kids and I knew how much fun it was having a family. Now I would never have a family of my own because of the treatment. And they were saying the chemotherapy was the only way I'd make it through.

"I was still working. I knew somehow that as long as I kept going I wouldn't die. You didn't die standing up. But it was getting harder and harder for me to put IVs into patients. The numbness and muscle stress were becoming more intense. I was put on the drug Elavil which helped with the nerve pain and muscle spasms. But there were many nights when I didn't sleep and I paced the floors of my studio apartment. My lifetime goal had been to become a physician, a healer, and no ugly old disease was going to stop me from attaining my goal of being the best doctor I could be. I kept thinking of what Dr. Osler had said about being a patient. I tried to be a good patient, a patient patient. I waited for MRI scans for hours. I was admitted to the hospital for chemotherapy in the afternoon, and the infusion wouldn't start until the next day. The physicians taking care of me were detached and impersonal. They treated me like a case study, not once acknowledging my depression or suggesting a support group. They never thought of anything they weren't taught in medical school. The focus was always on the disease.

"I knew I needed more if I was to go on and stop hurting. I looked into alternatives to conventional medicine to heal my spirit. I attended meetings at the Center for Attitudinal Healing in Tiburón, across the bay from San Francisco. I learned biofeedback to help with the muscle spasms. I tried acupuncture, but it wasn't effective for me. I had therapeutic massages at least twice a month and I started counseling. Through these meetings I met two other resident doctors at the University of California, San Francisco, both with critical cancer: a 33-year-old pediatric resident on a leave of absence with breast cancer, and John, a 29-year-old internal medicine resident who had a mesothelioma, a complication of radiation therapy he had had years before for Hodgkin's lymphoma. We took walks and compared notes as to how our fellow residents were treating us. I told John how one of my colleagues got upset when I left at 3:30 one Friday afternoon.

"'How do you get to split before the work is done?' he had said.

"I answered, 'I'd gladly stay if you'd go to the hospital and take my chemotherapy for me.' I had no takers.

"I remember, too, how irate my best friend was when I couldn't take Easter call for her because I was so sick with nausea and vomiting.

"John hadn't had the same experiences with the Internal Medicine residents. But his tumor was incurable and he died that year. So did the other resident with breast cancer."

Both deaths gave Bonnie much to think about and none of it was reassuring. She wondered about bad things happening in threes, but soon there were far more tangible concerns to deal with.

"Just when the chemotherapy appeared to be over my MRI showed a residual tumor necessitating more chemotherapy—six rounds more. 'If I can just make it through six more rounds, I'll be cured,' I told myself. I had no good veins left and the doctors recommended a porta cath, a portal implanted under the skin and attached to the subclavian vein under the collar bone. It looked like a third misplaced small breast and made me very self-conscious. Then my hair really started coming out in clumps from the chemotherapy, and my skin became this pale yellow color. I avoided looking in a mirror. At this point the other residents were getting angry because I wasn't taking calls and the cure was taking so long. Meetings with advisors and my department chief ensued. How could I possibly pay for all this treatment without a job and health insurance? We got paid $20,000 a year as residents. It was decided that I officially take no calls but continue to fulfill my duties on clinical rotations.

"There were some things on the positive side. I enjoyed the biofeedback and the visualizations, as a former creative artist with some considerable imagery. The biofeedback started to work and the nerve pain and muscle spasms abated a bit. Counseling was teaching me to move beyond denial and release the anger. The support groups, which I had latched on to, helped me to live day to day and to experience the release of living in the moment. Therapeutic massages were releasing the toxins in my body so that I could capitalize on the little energy I had left. However, the chemotherapeutic sessions had become more intense, and the violent vomiting retched every ounce of spirit from my cells."

There were radiation treatments as well. "Because of the encroachment of the tumor on my spinal cord, radiation was recommended after chemotherapy. Hadn't I had enough? I asked the doctors. No, we're going for the total cure, they responded. It sounded good. So, reluctantly now, I traveled to Stanford Medical Center and stayed a month, receiving 3400 Rads (radiation absorbed doses), a real good shot of radiation."

Since there was a good chance of recurrence within two years, Bonnie's doctors recommended a bone marrow harvest to remove some of her healthy bone marrow cells and freeze-dry them against a future need. Bonnie was devastated.

"Future need? I thought I would be cured. Had they been

lying to me the whole time? 'Yes,' they said. 'We wanted to get you through each course of treatment. But you should know you have this possibility of recurrence.'

"I took a deep breath, raised my head in prayer and cried alone. I went along with the bone marrow harvest. It was over on Thanksgiving. How appropriate, I thought: giving thanks to finally be over the treatment, giving a bone marrow harvest for that time when it might recur. My psyche might not have been so damaged if my doctors had been up-front with me from the onset."

And then Bonnie suffered an additional blow which had nothing to do with the medical therapy. Her boyfriend left her.

"My spirit might not have been so crushed if my boyfriend hadn't broken up with me at the termination of therapy, or if my fellow residents had been more supportive. But that Christmas, working at Children's Hospital in San Francisco, it hit me all at once. I truly became 'blue' with depression and I entertained thoughts of suicide. The hollow numbness which permeated every cell of my being was so overwhelming that I cracked. I couldn't go on any longer with the life I was living. I was plagued by uncertainty, living on the thin edge. I couldn't think straight. I notified my chief resident and the program director that I needed a leave of absence. My performance had been so poor it was readily granted.

"Here I was barely 30, just beginning my medical career, taking synthetic morphine tablets every night to get a few hours of troubled sleep, and not knowing how long it would be before they said nothing more could be done. I was a washout. I could see it plainly in the eyes of my colleagues. I was a goner. I had nowhere to turn.

"I'd heard of people going here and there, everywhere, looking for magical cures, but I had been in medical training too long to grasp at straws that provided false hope and then led to disenchantment.

"When I first heard of Dr. McGarey and her success in some cases of lymphoma, I was mildly interested. She had imposing credentials in the holistic field, which made sense to me as a young doctor. You not only treat the disease, but the whole person. I saw that in the emergency room and in the rounds I made. I saw how patients, critically ill, responded to a smile from a nurse or a doctor. So many patients with serious ailments, outside the parameters of cancer, remarkably recovered when they were continuously cheerful and optimistic. I wanted to know more about Gladys McGarey. I was told she looked on patients as friends and partners both in getting to the root of the problem, and in effecting a healing: in the psyche as well as in the physical self. Though I was a doctor in residence, without any vast practical experience, I knew enough to see that, however capable my doctors were, I was feeling no better. When a patient doesn't improve, he's not on his way to getting well. I decided I didn't have anything to lose. I discussed my options with my father, a doctor not wedded to any convention. He said with his usual wisdom that it was my life and that I was intelligent and sensitive enough to choose what was best for me. That helped me decide. I got on the phone and contacted the Scottsdale Holistic Medical Group in Arizona. It wasn't very often they had doctors as young as myself as patients."

Bonnie's parents had checked into my background and they were satisfied. They knew I was an allopathic physician, like Bonnie's father, *and* a homeopathic physician, combining the two disciplines in my holistic medical practice. I collaborated gladly with qualified conventional doctors of all specialties—surgeons, cardiologists, urologists, gynecologists, pediatricians and family practitioners.

The Griffiths looked around the clinic. They liked what they saw, but they felt a pang. It reminded them of the time they had taken their only daughter, a bright and eager freshman, to Mills College in Oakland. This was not the same, but they were as full of hope now as they were then and cheered by the friendly atmosphere.

Bonnie looked at me and knew she had come to the right place.

"Gladys took my hand, then hugged and kissed me, as though I were her daughter. All the tension left me. I felt as if I had come home."

My mind went back for a fleeting moment to my own training days. I looked into Bonnie's eyes and my heart went out to her. I saw in a glance what she had been through. She had been chemotherapied almost to death. She came to me as a frightened, sick young woman who had lost hope during the grueling experience she had been through. But she had a smile, though a trifle bleak, that let me know she had a sense of humor about herself. That was half the battle.

"The door to your health is wide open," I said, squeezing her hand. "You don't have to knock."

My physician eye looked beyond the confusion and depression, and saw from my own past the burgeoning physician within this young doctor. When Bonnie came to us, the entire focus of her previous medical therapy had been to kill the disease. Every thing, every thought had been directed towards death. The therapy was killing the cancer cells but it was also killing the healthy cells and her spirit. There was no thought of nurturing her as a total person. Her spirit and body were so beaten down that she had nothing to live for and no desire to live. Her will had been shaken, and the will, as we know, must always be supreme.

As Bonnie continued to work with biofeedback, her mind started to take hold and come alive. I could see her eyes brighten and occasionally there was a smile. I liked what I saw. I was looking at a young woman who could not yet see past the face of death. Our purpose was to turn her focus toward life. Her body needed loving care. Each cell had to be nurtured. Her mind needed to be stimulated and brought into the healing to control her body and let her know she was getting well. Her creative spirit needed to be encouraged and awakened. The physician within her had been on the edge of death and needed to take charge of her healing.

It was none too soon. No one had seen better than Bonnie just what she lacked. Throughout her travail, her physician within—and her own training—had been telling her she needed to be comforted and treasured, to feel the pulse of her body and the throb of her heart, to free her mind of sickness, and to frolic and play to her heart's content. She needed to be a young vibrant woman again: alive, excited and exciting.

She came out of the dregs, her dungeon of despair, in a matter of days. She describes it herself from the abyss of her resurging soul.

"My life had been on hold and anything to help me out of the pit of darkness in which I was engulfed was a godsend. My parents had flown with me to Arizona, petrified I might attempt to end it all. It was that bad. I was greeted with hugs, not only by Dr. Gladys, but by many of the patients. It almost bowled me over. I'll never forget that first day at the rehab center where the regeneration program was taking place. We were all given wonderfully colored sheets of chiffon and told to dance to the crescendo of classical music. I chose my color, blue, and felt the material, pulled it through my hands, slowly flung it in the air, and all of a sudden I was transformed into a ballerina twirling dizzily in the light . . . ah, the light! It was a bright sunny day in the Arizona desert in the middle of January, and all these strangers were dancing too. All of a sudden I had a vision of this mysterious woman with a light aura all around her. She beckoned us to form one huge circle and embrace one another.

Magically, I felt safe, nurtured and at peace for the first time in a year and a half. This, I thought to myself, would be my salvation, and indeed it was. For two weeks we immersed ourselves on a journey to see the light and get back in touch with the mind-body-spirit connection. There were a multitude of therapies to choose from: massage, colonics, meditation, diet, castor oil packs, Edgar Cayce remedies, group support and my favorite, art therapy. All those years of medical school and training hadn't afforded me the time to paint, sketch and express myself creatively. As a youngster I had remained 'in balance' by coupling my academic work with dance and art. What a revelation it was to realize my energy centers were misaligned because I hadn't been using them."

I, too, saw a new light in Bonnie's eyes. Her dreams changed, becoming more optimistic and hopeful, bright with the morning sunshine—no more midnight blues. I knew the physician within had come alive and was in charge. I could trust this inner "being" because I knew what Bonnie could do to bring about her own healing once she had something to fall back on—our support and that of the Lord we all prayed to.

After a week or two I had no more concerns. As a bright young doctor, able to analyze what had happened to her, I knew in time that Bonnie could reverse the process that had gotten her sick. I saw some dramatic changes take place on canvas. Her paintings, original in nature, captured her mood. Dark and somber at first, her work gradually became lighter, brighter, with depth. Where before she might have been hesitant, now she was daubing the canvas with swift, sure strokes. Her art showed a future full of life. Even her walk had changed. She was walking like she was going somewhere. And she was.

Bonnie was beginning to do things on her own, expressing her growing desire to get well. She began to take charge, and that brought back memories of what her three younger brothers used to call her as children—Miss Full Charge. The name lingered in her mind and deportment. She was doing it now, in this bruising fight to restore the flower of her youth.

Bonnie plunged into her painting. It had been her first ambition as a teenager. As she painted, she was producing healing alpha brain waves, promoting recovery.

"The thought blew my mind," Bonnie said. "Painting myself back to health. I would steal up to the art studio and let my creative juices flow. The symbolism of what I was creating with pastels was explained to me: my thymus, an energy center, had become congested (lymphoma) and my adrenal, another center, inactive. I learned so many tools in this experience I couldn't even begin to articulate them all. Some of the more salient teachings were: Forgive and forget. . . . let go. Don't live in the past because tomorrow is a new day. Forget the old traumas; bring them to the surface and dispel them forever.

"I rejoiced in this cancer that gave me a new life, this cancer that won't come back because I won't let it. The alpha waves of the biofeedback taught me to think of beautiful places like the beaches of Tahiti, with the warm waves caressing my soul, and to regain strength by visually being at one with other places close to nature—and God. I celebrated the power of affirmations. And I examined my life in light of my past. For example, was my residency what I really wanted, or was it what other people wanted for me? Many thoughts came to me. When we are not experiencing joy, we have forgotten to make peace of mind our single goal. We have become concerned about getting rather than giving. This peace is experienced as we learn to forgive the world and everyone in it and thereby see everyone, including ourselves, as blameless."

In reaching into the depths of her heart, soul and mind, Bonnie came up with an original concept, brought on by her continuing visualization of how she could bring about this inner peace she sought. She called it POPCORN, for the food she associated with the movies she had always liked. This unique concept was part of Bonnie's new creativity, a building of wellness out of sickness, and of wholeness out of the fragmented pieces of her life.

And what was POPCORN? The letters stood for: Positive attitude. Observation. Picture it. Concentrate. Organize. Review it. Natural environment.

"These were the tools, the thoughts, that kept me from killing myself and made me rejoice in life and living. The reentry to this new life wasn't easy. But I thought of Gladys and everyone else at the clinic, and I moved on. I transferred to the University of California at Davis, and I kept a promise I had made to Gladys just before I left that new Garden of Eden: If I wasn't truly happy being a radiologist after one more year, I would go back to being a general practice physician. And that's what happened."

We monitored Bonnie's progress after the Arizona experience. It didn't take her long to get into the swim. She started working at the County Clinics, then at an Urgent Care Facility. She is now an occupational physician. She had continued painting and has had several showings in Sacramento, making her home close by. She will never be alone. Her heart, which bore so much, is always open. While she can't have children, she does have a "little sister" who she is nurturing through adolescence with her mom, and loving it. After eight years she hasn't had the recurrence of cancer that all the doctors—except me—had predicted, thanks to the healthy shot of self-esteem and confidence she gave herself at the Arizona healing center.

The physician within had produced wonders for Bonnie in a few weeks. Friends who saw her only recently were struck by how radiantly healthy and happy she appeared. She bore no resemblance to the young medical resident who had had to constantly fight a gnawing, heartrending pain while brooding over the cancer eating away at her body. Now, there was no more cancer and no more fear. Instead, there was a new role as a compassionate healer who remembered what it was like to be a patient.

"Yes," Bonnie wrote recently, "it's wonderful to be alive and well, helping people who are ill, instead of being obsessed by my own illness as I strive to carry on with my duties as a doctor. I have a new outlook, a new empathy. I look beyond the patients' illnesses to the kind of people they are and to the needs they have, above and beyond those necessitated by their illness. I find it uplifting to help them triumph over their sickness, to reach deep within themselves in the healing partnership we share. There is no separation or boundary between us, just as there was none between me and Gladys McGarey. I shall always remember and treasure her for what she taught me as she was saving my life: to have faith and persevere; to love for love's sake; to count my blessings on the darkest day when my heart quivers with fear and my legs tremble. Gladys helped me to understand that the God who put us here, who stands for love, will listen if we rise to the challenge he has given us and we strive to make this a more caring world, any way we can. We just need to do our best with what we have, where we are."

Life Is a Passing Through

*Death is but the beginning
of life. The passing in,
the passing out.*

—Edgar Cayce

I loved Stella as a patient. I loved her as a woman. And she was a woman first and foremost. She was able to give more, even with all her ailments, and perhaps because of them. Stella loved every moment of her life. She lived with humor and joy, and could laugh in the midst of pain. She had no fear of dying, for she believed there was no death. She spoke often of the angels who hovered over her bedside when she was most stricken and thought to be dying. Yet she always rallied, brought back by a brave heart and the knowledge that it was not yet her time to go to that other place. That was how she thought of death—that other place, where she could discuss Plato, Aristotle and all the wonderful masters of ancient Greece, with the father she treasured.

Stella had no doubts about this other place. Her angels, like her father, described it to her. It was a place of total communication, and a sharing of all that was good and undying. She felt her father's presence, and in meditation, communicated with him. He was his wise old self, patient and endearing, telling her when she spoke of going on that there was more for her to do, more for her to be. She needed to let the younger people know, particularly, that you moved on in God's time, but lived in your own, and you moved on with hope and expectation, not despair.

"There are angels and souls on the other side who guide us," Stella would say, and her belief made it so for her. "I firmly believe that the physical body dies, but the soul lives on. These angels I've seen are very real. As real as the sickness I've known, as real as my husband and daughter and the physician within who cured the cancer and gangrene the doctors in New York called incurable."

Stella came to me as a patient asking for help but soon became a friend and a teacher. Although she was sick she radiated health. Her body may have been in trouble, but her spirit never wavered. I marveled as I watched her overcome asthma, then the lymphoma and gangrene, grateful that she could walk and drive, even dance, and that her prosthesis fit so well. Many years later she would face lymphoma again, this time with a chronically defective heart, and she would win that fight, too. I don't know how many times she looked death in the face and said, "Not now, my work isn't done. I don't have a grandchild yet." And death walked away as Stella came back to us.

"My heart won't let me down before I'm ready," she'd say, "and I won't be ready until my angels come and take me."

One priceless ingredient—love—brought Stella through the

dark days in New York when they chipped away at one leg, and were planning to take the other, while saying they could hold out no hope for her unless she took chemotherapy for her lymphoma. She was spared by the love of her family, the love of her friends, and her own love for them and anyone else who needed her love.

She turned to her husband George, always a staunch support, and said evenly, "George, am I going to die?"

"No, Stella," he said, putting his arm around her.

"Are you sure, George?" she said without a tremor.

He smiled. "I'm sure. I won't let you die."

She said, "No thanks" to the chemotherapy—and kept her leg.

She made a positive thing of her experience with the physicians in New York. She had nothing but praise and love for their conscientious efforts to save her life. "They were doing what they'd been trained to do."

So with the love that got her through her illness, a proud Stella returned to the New York hospital to share her triumph with the doctors and nurses there. A nurse asked if she would give a class on alternative medicine and our wonderful Stella became an emissary for the holistic approach in medicine. She said it as well as or better than I could, for she had been through more and her physician within was speaking as a patient. She saw her illness as an adventure in consciousness and a time to grow. She was the best example of it. On two more visits to the hospital, at the request of its staff, she gave classes in relaxing with biofeedback, and in color therapy for relieving stress.

Everyone at our clinic was struck by her courage and discipline as she kept on with her visualizations and her diet. We felt her love as she embraced us with her warm smile and soft voice. How wonderfully she touched our lives with her presence. She lived with pain and at times fear—for she was very human—but she never allowed herself to be stuck in the dark valley of hopelessness. Drawing on her reservoir of courage, she came out of it smiling and full of hope, a word that speaks deeply of Stella. She was always ready to help others who were facing hard places to have hope because it had meant so much to her. She valued her husband's quiet support, and rejoiced in her daughter Athena's happy marriage. When a grandson was born, she saw her dream come true: the continuity of life reenacted in this life, and the harbinger of a new life for her.

She had no doubt about it. The spirit of immortality was in her veins. During childhood she had breathed in those wonderful stories of the Greeks of ancient times—Hercules and Apollo—immortalized in life and death. She could laugh and say, "I'm no Hercules," but the image stuck, fostered by a Christian belief that death is but a beginning.

She had her low spots, but her humor invariably would brim to the surface. Settling into the Phoenix-Scottsdale area for her battle for life, she laughed and said, "I shall rise like Phoenix from the ashes."

As she healed she developed an inner peace and serenity. Friends marveled that she appeared to look younger, the result, in some ways, of a better diet and a new inner strength. It pleased her that she wasn't slipping away into old age. I could never think of Stella as being old, for she had a lively interest in everything around her, especially children, with their keen insight into adults.

"Stay with the young in heart as much as you can," she'd say. "It's contagious."

Stella passed away months after this book was wrapped up— but not completed. This book could never be complete without the rest of Stella's story.

Her daughter was at her bedside when Stella moved on. Athena, an only child, was inconsolable. She missed the warmth and comfort of their daily conversations, and the love so constant it had a life of its own. The day after her mother's death Athena got into her car and drove around aimlessly, just to be moving, to be doing something. She came to a stop at the home of a psychic who was her mother's friend. As the psychic came to the door, Athena cried, "Is my mother all right? Is she happy? Is she with people she loves?"

The psychic, Linda Madrini, had been expecting her. She pondered a moment, then said without any preamble, "Athena, please give me time to contact your mother. I will let you know if anything comes through."

She called the next morning. Athena leaped to the phone. "Yes?" It was all she could say.

"Athena," the sensitive said, "don't shed another tear. Your mother is very happy and free, and joyfully reunited with her father. She said she will be your little boy's guardian angel. When you see him quietly staring into the sky, know that he is listening to your mother. She will be expressing her love for him. She has not left any of you."

Shortly after her mother's death, Athena began to feel Stella's presence whenever there was a need of any kind in the family. "I know for sure," she said, "that my mother guards my child and is there for him.

"Sometimes Steven will stop playing, sit up erect in his crib, lift his eyes and appear to be listening. A thrill goes through me as I realize my mother is singing to him an old Greek lullaby, 'Kuña Bella' (loosely, 'Beautiful Baby in a Cradle'), as she sang to me when I was a child. And little Steven will point to a picture of Stella and smile, saying *'Yiayia,'* which is 'grandmother' in Greek."

Stella will forever be a prime example and inspiration for our medical practice. She was never too busy to sit down and discuss her trials in overcoming illness, never too busy to pat a dog on the head or kiss a child. "Love is the best medicine of all," she would say, "and don't forget to love yourself." It was a home recipe she lived with and it moved on with her and her unquenchable spirit.

Athena is in the mold of her mother. And like her mother, who believed in the angels who communed with her at her bedside, Athena believes these same angels are now with her and her boy. And who is to say these angels aren't very real, when, as is known, with an open mind—and an open heart—anything can happen.

As a physician who believes that death is an unfinished part of life, I have no trouble helping the dying to move more easily on their way. Birth and death are the two things common to everyone in this universe. As the great Russian novelist and philosopher Tolstoy told his grieving daughter: "Don't mourn for me. Life is a passing through. Death is the reality—and the Promise."

ADDENDUM

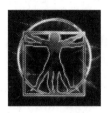

You've often heard it said: "An ounce of prevention is worth a pound of cure." Even insurance companies recognize the value of preventive medicine, allowing for periodic checkups to the doctor as a way to ultimately cut costs (and, incidentally, save lives). The concept has permeated all medical disciplines, but preventive medicine goes beyond seeing a doctor and getting a physical. It involves taking a few precautionary measures to ensure a sound body, mind and spirit. Below are some tangible steps you can take to consciously improve your life, regardless of whether or not you currently face a health challenge. If you "obey" these commandments, you will surely lead a more fulfilling life, and that, in itself, may prevent you from becoming "dis-eased."

The 10 Commandments
of Wholeness

1. Be positive. Give yourself something to live for. So many illnesses are born of the mind. What we think is so often what we become. When a body is truly diseased or ill, there are usually many things wrong with it. But there is an essential part of the body which is still functional and capable of turning things around with the proper incentive. It is so much easier to contact the physician within and turn a sickness around when you have a burning desire to get well. When World War II abruptly ended with the surrender of Japan, a lot of sick people, bedridden, critically ill, got out of their hospital beds, threw on their clothes and streamed out of the hospital. "Sick, how can I be sick," one woman cried, "when my boy will be coming home after five years of me worrying myself to death?"

2. Love yourself, without being indulgent. You are the center of your universe. Unless you keep that center strong you cannot help anyone—including yourself. Even a locomotive can pull only so many cars. I have worked with families where the caregivers completely devoted their time and energy to caring for other members of the family and neglected their own well-being. Sometimes they became so run-down that they died before the sick relatives they had cared for. These caregivers had never given the physician within themselves a chance. They had forgotten the "self" in the biblical injunction, "Love your neighbor as yourself."

3. Be forgiving. My mother, a physician for more than 60 years, used to say, "There is so much good in the worst of us and so much bad in the best of us that it hardly behooves us to put down the rest of us." In the absence of forgiveness we have malice and judgment, which tend to put a strain on mind and body, deplete the spirit and lead to disease and premature aging. My forgiving patients so often look ages younger than their years. They are easy on themselves as well as others. This easiness becomes a way of life and is good for the arteries. Some, in their 80s, go bicycling. Others, in their 90s, walk a mile daily. They are the survivors of this world.

4. Keep your life balanced. We are multidimensional. The metaphysician Edgar Cayce said, "Spirit is the life, the mind the builder, the physical the result." If any aspect of your person is overemphasized, it's likely that the other aspects are slighted. Too much time given to rapt thought may deprecate the body and spirit, bringing an imbalance in life. A flabby Elvis Presley, enamored of yoga, told Daya Mata, the head of the Yoga Self-Realization Center in Los Angeles, that he wanted to give up his singing career and become a monk in her order. She told him that yoga was a blend of the physical, mental and spiritual, and that he could serve best by getting himself in shape physically, cutting out junk foods and turning to spiritual music. He listened in part, and made the album *How Great Thou Art,* a tribute to the Lord which inspired millions. Unfortunately, he continued with his junk food, stayed overweight and came to an untimely end.

5. Take time to meditate and pray. In meditation you listen to God. In prayer you talk to God. Both practices bolster your connection with the universal world. You need to give yourself some quiet time and get to know your physician within. Pray for love. With love you fill the emptiness within you and strengthen your faith in yourself. This faith allows us to grow. It may not move mountains, but it moves people.

Love also instills courage and fosters serenity. It keeps your blood pressure down and your spirits up. It lets you do more than you thought you could and be greater than you think you are. Without love there is no real healing—a healing that reaches deep into the spirit. The physician within responds to that love, which transforms the ordinary into the extraordinary and the common into the divine. The physician within is always there for you.

6. Listen closely to whatever message your body has for you. Use common sense and take care of your body—it is the only one you have. If humanly possible, you should exercise every day, if only for 10 or 15 minutes. Whatever your age you need to keep your body firm and resilient. You are as old as your bones say you are. There's an old saying, "A wheat field which is green and alive bends when the wind blows, but when it is dry and the wind blows, it breaks." You need to keep the circulation moving in your body. The blood and lymph bring nourishment and strength to your bones. Without exercise, a brittleness of the bones, osteoporosis, becomes a geriatric problem no matter what drugs you take to prevent it. Your bones need the push and pull of flexible muscles to keep them from drying out like the wheat field. Keep exercising. There's nothing like yoga to keep the muscles supple.

7. Look for humor and joy in every situation. Laugh and the world laughs with you. Cry and you cry alone. We all know something of the wisdom of this saying, perhaps without realizing that the joy of laughter and the gift of humor are indispensable to our health. Laughter stimulates the adrenals and activates the immune system. So many people I know are burdened with problems—financial, family, health. Yet they are able to deal with them because they find humor and joy in their lives—in the smile of a child, the supportive love of family and friends. Ask the Lord for help, and he will give you strength. Out of life's trials comes the opportunity for growth. Growth brings a new appreciation of self and others—a new clarity of mind and body, and a new wholeness.

8. Breathe deeply. We can live without food for three or four weeks, without water for three or four days. But we can't live without oxygen—the breath of life—for more than

three or four minutes as a rule. There is nothing more important to our well-being than the air we breathe. A great teacher
of yoga, 100 years young, was asked by a student what physical exercise or posture was of the most importance. She
smiled and said, "The breathing." As you exercise, you concentrate on the breathing. Visualizing as you breathe, breathe
in health and breathe out illness. Breathe in hope and breathe
out fear. Breathe in love and breathe out anger. Before you
know it, your body and mind are responding. You'll feel as if
you are walking on air. And you will be. Your blood will be
pulsing through your veins and you will be bursting with
energy, ready to take on the world.

9. Dream yourself to health. Tell yourself that you will
dream when you retire for the night. Soon you will be having
dreams significant to your health and well-being. You must
write the dreams down right away or they will dematerialize
as though in thin air. It is amazing how the physician within
guides the sleeping patient's subconscious mind into problem
areas that their conscious mind has been grappling with.

10. Know that healing comes from within. You do it
all the time without thinking about it. You cut your finger.
The blood flows, cleansing the wound. Then the blood coagulates, forming a scab which protects the underlying wound.
When the wound is completely healed, the scab falls off by
itself. If you think of this at all, you think of it as something
that is perfectly natural. And it is. Every cell in the body has
an innate intelligence of its own, responsive to the body's
subconscious impulse to heal. This automatic response can
be reproduced anywhere in the body by giving the patient
access to the physician within. There is nothing mysterious
or subtle about this process. The subconscious mind directs

the healing alpha brain waves to the diseased cells. I have seen it work a thousand times. All it takes is faith and fortitude, and an open mind.

THE GLADYS TAYLOR McGAREY MEDICAL FOUNDATION

A pioneer in the holistic health field, Dr. Gladys Taylor McGarey established the Gladys Taylor McGarey Medical Foundation in 1989 as a resource for wellness education and a legacy to help emerging health-care professionals carry the art of healing into the 21st century.

A non-profit organization, the foundation has been a leader in advocating the integration of the best of holistic and conventional medicines. This is now called integrative medicine and includes a rebirth of practices that were part of ancient healing traditions used by people around the world. Rather than just treating disease, the focus of medicine is shifting to maintaining good health and preventing illness.

Through its educational programs for the general public and health care professionals, the foundation is dedicated to: advancing human understanding of the body-mind-spirit relationship in healing; encouraging wellness and wholeness through the combination of the best of conventional and holistic medical practices; and serving as a model for education, research and the application of integrative healing practices. The foundation publishes an award-winning newsletter, *HealthLinks,* sponsors study groups for physicians, holds workshops and seminars, and facilitates Dr. McGarey's lectures and educational projects.

The foundation is partnering with a major medical center to develop a preceptorship in alternative medicine for medical students, and plans a fellowship program in holistic medicine for physicians who want to add the art of medicine to the science, which they are already practicing.

The ultimate goal of the foundation is to establish an international healing center. Dr. McGarey's dream is to create a state-of-the-art integrative medical facility that combines the best of holistic and conventional practices. This facility will serve as a global classroom, via telecommunications, where medical experts can share knowledge as medicine evolves to face the challenges of improving health in the next millennium.

Both the general public and health-care professionals are encouraged to use the Gladys Taylor McGarey Medical Foundation as a resource for health and wellness information. The work of the foundation is supported solely by donations and volunteers. We welcome your support as we work to improve the health of this and future generations.

For more information about the foundation, please call or write:

Gladys Taylor McGarey Medical Foundation
7350 East Stetson Drive, Suite 208
Scottsdale, Arizona 85251
(602) 946-4544 • fax (602) 946-6902

ABOUT THE AUTHORS

Dr. Gladys Taylor McGarey is internationally known for her pioneering work in holistic medicine, the physician-patient partnership and natural birthing. She has practiced medicine for 50 years and has advocated a holistic approach to patient care through her worldwide lectures and writing. In 1992, she was one of 100 physicians and researchers appointed to the National Institutes of Health's (NIH) newly created Office of Alternative Medicine. A founding member and past president of the American Holistic Medical Association, she is currently president of the Arizona Board of Homeopathic Medical Examiners, a director of the American Board of Holistic Medicine, and member of the Advisory Board of the Institute for Natural Healing.

Considered a visionary in holistic health, she mentored many leaders in the current global movement embracing alternative medicine modalities. Her work through the not-for-profit Gladys Taylor McGarey Medical Foundation helps to expand the knowledge and application of holistic principles and the integration of holistic and conventional medicines through educational programs for both the medical profession and the general public. In addition to numerous papers and articles, she authored the book *Born to Live,* and coauthored *There Will Your Heart Be Also.*

Born and raised in India, the daughter of American medical missionaries, Dr. McGarey came to the United States at the age of 16 to attend college. She graduated from Women's Medical College in Philadelphia, Pennsylvania, in 1946. She and her former husband practiced medicine in Wellsville, Ohio, before moving to Phoenix, Arizona, in 1955, where they later cofounded the A.R.E. Clinic. She raised her six children while maintaining an active medical practice. Her children are now in the fields of family practice medicine, orthopedic surgery, pediatrics, physical therapy, counseling and the ministry.

She blended her knowledge of Eastern and Western medicine to help patients who came from throughout the world. Dr. McGarey educated people about the mind-body-spirit connection in healing and began speaking internationally at numerous holistic health symposiums. She was among a small group of professional women chosen to tour the People's Republic of China and pioneered the first acupuncture training session for physicians in the United States in 1972.

Today, Dr. McGarey continues to work as a family physician with her daughter, Helene Wechsler, M.D., M.D.(H), at the Scottsdale Holistic Medical Group, a family medical practice they founded in 1989.

Dr. McGarey helped launch the natural childbirth movement in the United States. As an innovator in the natural birthing movement, Dr. McGarey founded the widely acclaimed Baby Buggy Program in 1978. The program featured a fully-equipped paramedical vehicle that accompanied a certified nurse-midwife to all home deliveries, standing by to take mother and baby to the hospital in case of an emergency. She was a leader in childbirth education and, during the early 1970s, was one of the first physicians to support the rights of obstetrical patients to have their husbands present in the delivery room.

A much-honored "true physician," Dr. McGarey has been

called the "Mother of Holistic Medicine" by her peers, and is considered a dear family friend by the many thousands of patients she literally embraces and to whom she has unselfishly given of her time and energy for over half a century.

Jess Stearn is an award-winning author and a celebrated journalist. He was a prizewinning reporter for the *New York Daily News* and won the Silurian Award, given by the city's top editors, for his series on crime in the schools. This series, which added 300,000 readers to the newspaper's circulation, broke the payola scandal involving pay-as-you-play disk jockeys and resulted in a U.S. Senate investigation. As an editor at *Newsweek,* Stearn won the Newspaper Guild Front Page Award for outstanding journalism for a cover story on Joseph Kennedy, father of President John F. Kennedy.

He is the author of over 30 books, several of which were best-sellers, including: *Soulmates; Yoga, Youth and Reincarnation; Door to the Future; The Sixth Man; I Judas; The Power of Alpha Thinking; The Search for the Soul: Psychic Lives of Taylor Caldwell; Prophet in His Own Country;* and the #1 *New York Times* bestseller, *Edgar Cayce: The Sleeping Prophet.*